Person-Centred Teams

Person-Centred Teams

A Practical Guide to
Delivering Personalisation
Through Effective Team-work

HELEN SANDERSON AND MARY BETH LEPKOWSKY

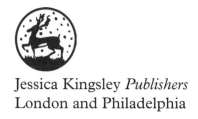

Jessica Kingsley *Publishers*
London and Philadelphia

First published in 2014
by Jessica Kingsley Publishers
73 Collier Street
London N1 9BE, UK
and
400 Market Street, Suite 400
Philadelphia, PA 19106, USA

www.jkp.com

Library of Congress Cataloging in Publication Data
A CIP catalog record for this book is available from the Library of Congress

British Library Cataloguing in Publication Data
A CIP catalogue record for this book is available from the British Library

ISBN 978 1 84905 455 3
eISBN 978 0 85700 830 5

Printed and bound in Great Britain by Bell and Bain Ltd, Glasgow

Contents

Acknowledgements

Helen and Mary Beth have been working together over the past five years to create and test the current model of person-centred teams and to build a community of practice around these ideas. This book builds on and shares our earlier learning around developing person-centred teams. This started with Helen's PhD which focused on person-centred planning, organisational development and person-centred teams. The work was further developed with colleagues in HSA, in particular, Ruth Gorman, Jo Harvey, Amanda George and Michelle Livesley, and then with Stephen Stirk from United Response.

The learning shared in this book reflects the work of the Learning Community for person-centred practices. You can learn more about their work at www.learningcommunity.us.

'Positive and Productive Meetings' were originally developed by Helen Sanderson, Amanda George and Marc Archambault.

Thank you to Julie Barclay for her design of the graphics used throughout the book.

Mary Beth Lepkowsky

Heartfelt appreciation goes to my friend and co-author, Helen Sanderson, for her clarity of vision and excitement about sharing our message. Without her patience and encouragement this collaboration would not have been possible.

I am deeply grateful for those who applied these practices and spoke of their significant impact on team development, effectiveness and outcomes. In particular I thank friends and colleagues from Tri-Counties Regional Center (TCRC) including the Oxnard Children's Team, San Luis Obispo Adult Team, Santa Barbara Children's Team, Oxnard Early Start Team, Organizational Development Team and Director's Team. Thanks also to the Luis Oasis Senior Center, Santa Ynez Valley Humane Society, ARCA Training and Information Group, Star Choices of Georgia, NorthStar Supported Living Services, PathPoint Inc. and Channel Island Social Services.

To celebrate TCRC staff, who give tirelessly in support of others, Mary Beth is donating her author royalties to the Tri-Counties Regional Center Help Fund to assist persons with developmental disabilities and their families in emergency situations when there is no other source of financial assistance.

Helen Sanderson

Thank you to the following people and organisations who shared their learning, stories and examples within this book.

Dr Samuel Crawshaw, Gill Goodwin, Rowan Hall, Certitude, Sanchi Murison, Dimensions, Real Life Options, Borough Care Ltd and Bruce Lodge, Andy Gitsham, Positive Futures, Howard Bousfield, Michelle Livesley, Mary Lou Bourne, Jon Ralphs, Tim Parr, Vicky Jones, Enable Southwest in Western Australia, Cheryl Swan, Tracey Bush, United Response, Gill Bailey, Friends of the Elderly, Ruth Gorman, Amanda George, Julie Malette, Jo Harvey and Charlotte Sweeney.

Finally, thank you to Mary Beth for being a wonderful thinking partner.

Preface

This is the third book in a collection of titles about using person-centred practices with individuals, teams and organisations. Our main purpose in writing it was to share what we have been trying and learning about what person-centred practices look like when they're used with staff as well as people who use services.

The people we had in mind when we were writing this book typically have responsibility for helping a team work well together. Although team leaders are mainly addressed within the context of *Person-Centred Teams*, we hope it has a much broader appeal.

The process of learning about person-centred teams grew through our partnership with Michael Smull, and the work of the Learning Community for Person-Centred Practices, and then applying it to teams. Our writing started with the first version of our person-centred team manual that was part of our training in 2004 with Jo Harvey and Ruth Gorman.

Amanda George, Michelle Livesley and Stephen Stirk helped update the manual in 2009, and it was soon afterwards that we started to develop this current version of *Person-Centred Teams*.

Throughout the chapters we share stories and examples from our own teams and teams we have worked with. You'll read about teams in schools, health services and community and non-profit sectors, as well as teams supporting people with mental health issues, learning disabilities and dementia. These are examples from areas that we have worked in and we hope that you can see how you could apply these principles and ideas creatively to your setting. While issues and context may differ, the factors that challenge teams and the strategies that strengthen them are universal.

If you want to read more about how person-centred practices deliver personalisation with individuals, you might find *A Practical Guide to Delivering Personalisation: Person-Centred Practice in Health and Social Care* useful (Sanderson and Lewis 2011). If you are interested in how person-centred practices can be used in organisations, you might be interested in *Creating Person-Centred Organisations* (Stirk and Sanderson 2012).

We sincerely appreciate you joining us on our journey of discovery and we hope that the content contained within *Person-Centred Teams* will help you discover your own path to becoming a positive and productive team leader.

Introduction

> Everyone wants to work in an engaging, exciting workplace...research shows consistently that happier, more engaged employees are more productive. We know, intuitively, that a workplace where people come first is the workplace we want to be part of.
>
> *Professor Julian Birkinshaw (London Business School)[1]*

Ask yourself the following questions:

- What does it feel like to be a member of your team?

- Do you feel energised and motivated to produce quality work?

- Do you feel trusted, have clear guidelines and freedom to produce innovative ideas?

- Do you feel recognised and supported by the people around you?

If you answered yes to any or all of these questions, you are among the 21 per cent of staff members who feel fully engaged at work. Only 21 per cent of staff members in an organisation feel they are 100 per cent engaged in their work.[2]

Workplace experts Marcus Buckingham and Curt Coffman headed a research study conducted by Gallup, Inc. involving 80,000 managers across different industries. In their acclaimed book, *First, Break All the Rules: What the World's Greatest Managers Do Differently*, Buckingham and Coffman identified 12 questions that correlate with attaining, keeping and measuring employee satisfaction.[3]

1. Do I know what's expected of me at work?

2. Do I have the materials and equipment I need to do my work right?

3. At work, do I have the opportunity to do what I do best every day?

4. In the last seven days have I received recognition or praise for doing good work?

5. Does my supervisor, or someone at work, seem to care about me as a person?

6. Is there someone at work who encourages my development?

7. Do my opinions seem to count at work?

8. Does the mission/purpose of my company make me feel my job is important?

9. Are my co-workers committed to doing quality work?

10. Do I have a best friend at work?

11. In the last six months has someone at work talked to me about my progress?

12. This last year have I had opportunities at work to learn and to grow?

Person-Centred Teams was written for team leaders – who are the hub of an organisation's success – to help them elevate the strength and level of commitment among staff to work brilliantly together and to achieve success. We share person-centred thinking tools and practices to build a purposeful person-centred team plan that will make it more likely that staff can answer 'yes' to the 12 fundamental questions above.

What does 'person-centred team' mean?

Person-centred teams focus on interpersonal work relationships to deliver a culture of superior performance, trust, engagement and accountability based on the tenet that if one fails…all fail.

The term 'person-centred team' may be new to you – you will not find the term 'person-centred team' in the business literature. Person-centred teams bring together the concept of high-performing teams, the values of person-centred counselling developed by Carl Rogers, and person-centred practices. Person-centred teams provide a focus on people and relationships, to deliver great performance together and use a range of person-centred practices to achieve this.

The original concept of person-centred teams was based on the Drexler/Sibbet[4] Team Performance Model adapted from six years of researching human services, and then integrating that data with person-centred practices.

Person-centred practices are a range of thinking tools and approaches developed by Michael Smull and The Learning Community (www.learningcommunity.us), reinforced by the concept that people need to understand what is 'important to' and 'important for' someone, and to find a balance between the two. 'Important to' is what really matters to the person, what makes their life meaningful, and what they want to have present in their work and home life. 'Important for' relates to what must happen for a person to remain healthy and safe, and what other people need to know or do to enable the person to function at their best. It is crucial that team managers understand this.

Research suggests that employees tend to leave organisations due to a poor relationship with their manager. The Chartered Management Institute in the UK found that 49 per cent of staff would be willing to take a pay cut if it meant working with a more supportive, team-orientated manager (HR Review, 11 November 2009, p.117):

> The impact of a manager's behaviour is believed to be more essential than other employee-focused initiatives. If (your manager) sets clear expectations, knows you, trusts you, and invests in you, then you can forgive the company its lack of profit sharing programme. It is better to work for a great manager in an old fashioned company than for a terrible manager in a company offering an enlightened, employee-focused culture.[5]

The particular focus of our work is with teams working in health, social care, education and the voluntary sector. In each of these areas in the UK, there is a drive towards personalisation, to make sure that people are at the centre of decisions about their lives and services, and have as much choice and control as possible. In the United States, this is reflected in the term 'person-centred services'; in Canada 'person-directed support'; and in Australia 'person-centred support'. No matter its designation, effective personalisation must be delivered by person-centred staff and teams across the entire organisation.

Why are person-centred teams important to delivering personalised or person-centred services?

In *Creating Person-Centred Organisations* we argued that you needed to have a person-centred organisation in order to deliver person-centred services and personalisation. We suggested that personalisation requires transformation in the ways that organisations, and therefore teams, work.

A person-centred organisation has people at its heart – both people it serves and people it employs. This impacts on the whole organisation's processes and structures, and transforms the traditional organisational hierarchy, putting decision-making as close to people supported as possible. The DNA of a person-centred team and organisation is using person-centred practices to deliver its vision and values.

You cannot manage a team in a traditional, hierarchical way and expect team members to deliver truly personalised, person-centred support to individuals. Therefore, we need to explore how teams can work together differently, and productively, so that the values of personalisation and person-centred work can be seen and felt in all aspects of how an organisation works. Personalisation requires a person-centred culture throughout organisations, and this book describes what this means at a team level.

What would you see in a person-centred team?

In person-centred teams, people are central – both the people supported by the team and the people in it. If your team makes products, rather than provides services, this is just as important, in relation to thinking about your customers and your staff. This is what you would see in a person-centred team.

Person-centred teams:

- have a shared sense of purpose, know what success means in relation to their purpose, know why they are there, and why their work matters

- know what is important to their members, and how to support members individually and collectively

- allocate roles and tasks based on members' strengths and interests

- reflect regularly on what their members are doing and learning so they can continuously develop and improve

- maintain a 'living record' of who the team is, their purpose, how people work together, what they are working towards, and how they are doing this – a person-centred team plan.

There are five elements to a person-centred team – Purpose, People, Performance, Process and Progress – and two thought-provoking questions need to be asked of each:

Purpose

- Why are we here?

- Why am I part of this team?

People

- Who are we?

- How do we support one another?

Performance

- What does success look like?

- How can we know how well we are doing?

Process

- How will we work together?

- How will we deliver success?

Progress

- How are we doing?

- How can we improve?

The goal of a person-centred team is not merely to get along, but rather to get aligned, and, through that, to get results. Performance is aligned with delivering purpose: the processes that the team use are the ones most likely to deliver performance and reflect what matters to people. Progress starts with how you are doing in delivering your performance.

We have been thinking about what 'performance' and 'progress' mean for us in the context of writing this book. Success for us is about sharing learning and growing a community of practice around these ideas, and this book is one way towards this. In this book we take you step-by-step through purpose, people, performance, process and progress and, for each, give you a range of ways to choose from and a means to check how you are doing. At the end, in the conclusion, we offer you three ways to get started in a day.

Chapter 1

Profiles and Plans

One-page profiles and person-centred team plans are living records of team members and how the team work together. In this chapter we lay the foundation for the rest of the book by introducing one-page profiles and how they are used in organisations. (If you're already familiar with person-centred planning, a team plan is the equivalent.)

Have you ever participated in a team-building day or retreat? Although they can be brilliant for creating a feeling of cohesion and well-being, the afterglow of bonding can fade – and seldom do people think about recording the sessions to utilise back at the workplace. A person-centred team plan is a place to record what you learn about each other, why you are together in a team and how you agree to work together.

When Helen worked as an occupational therapist in a hospital, she was asked to read the procedures manual within the first three days (there were 185 pages!). When she started work with a local authority, there was no procedures manual; instead there was a series of forms to be completed, and the manager sat down and explained each form in turn. A person-centred team plan introduces you to a team, who they are and how they work together. It is the best of a personalised procedures manual (but briefer!) and clarifies the core expectations (which may include what forms to complete) as well as where you can use your judgement and be creative. It also gives you a head start on getting to know the individuals in the team – through a one-page profile you can learn the equivalent of a day away team-building, or three evenings out socialising with team members.

As previously mentioned, the forthcoming chapters show how person-centred practices can be used to address the five aspects of a person-centred team: purpose, people, performance, process and progress. The outcomes from exploring these areas are recorded in the person-centred team plan that serves as a road map to achieving goals while honouring what's important to team members.

There is a bewildering array of team-building exercises and processes. A quick internet search will give you over a hundred books or exercises to choose from, all potentially useful. We think that you will have a greater impact and make better use of team-building resources when exercises are designed to gain insights about working together and the information is recorded for ongoing use by the team, in a person-centred team plan. This plan often begins with one-page profiles, so let's start by taking a closer look at these.

One-page profiles

A one-page profile – as the name infers – is a concise summary of who a person is on one page. It's different from a biography or resume in that it captures who the person is now and does not cover past career-related activities. A one-page profile typically has three sections – an appreciation about the person; what is important to them from their perspective; and how to support them well. In some situations it is useful to add an additional section, either around history or future, and we share an example of that later in this chapter. Don't try to make it a one-size-fits-everything page – we recommend that you keep to the three headings and only include history or future if this is required for how you are going to use the information – back to 'purpose' again. If you just want a page with a variety of different headings, that's fine, but it is not a one-page profile.

One-page profiles are the building blocks for developing a more comprehensive person-centred team plan, which includes details about the team purpose, team members, standards of performance, agreements about working together, team goals and actions.

It is not a new form to fill in. One-page profiles are developed through conversations and using person-centred thinking tools, for example, talking about good days and bad days. They provide information about what is important to you, and how you need to be supported. We look at these in the People chapter. A good one-page profile will make you feel as if you have met the person, even before you meet them. The amount of detail is crucial. They can also be solely work focused (like Mary Beth's profile, Figure 1.1) or broader, covering all areas of a person's life (like Helen's profile, Figure 1.2).

Dr Samuel Crawshaw, Head of Year at the Manchester Grammar School, describes how he started to develop his own one-page profile, and was then supported to add detail by Gill, a trainer with Helen Sanderson Associates (HSA), who asked him questions to help draw out the information to complete his one-page profile:

> After our pastoral school staff spoke to Helen about how other schools had been using one-page profiles, we realised that the first step in introducing them to our pupils would be for teachers to have a go at writing their own. My first attempt at writing anything down was at home during the summer holidays. I asked my wife and children for some attributes to put in the appreciation box on my one-page profile. My daughter said that I was 'not boring' while my wife suggested that I was a 'great dancer'. My thoughts on what is important to me were quite vague, which meant that I struggled to fill in the final box describing how others could support me.
>
> At that stage this was the information I had in my one-page profile:

Like and admire

Friendly, organised, not boring, great dancer.

What is important to me

- I like supporting my family and making sure they are okay.

- I love watching good (and bad) films with my kids.

- Running.

- Playing with my guinea pigs, Nibbles and Pops.

- Experiencing wilderness.

- Making biology inspiring.

one page profile

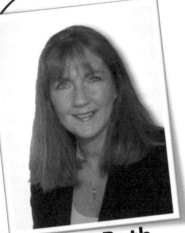

Mary Beth

What others appreciate about me

visionary
creative
leader
considerate
talented

What is important to me

- To feel connected to my community and workplace
- To believe my work is making a lasting impact
- To be part of a team with a shared goal
- To have a schedule, but not a repetitive routine. I like change.
- To have time to work independently as well as with others
- To engage in big picture, strategy discussions
- To create visually engaging, interactive and practical training
- To balance work & family and be home for Friday family movie nights
- To have a flexible schedule and ability to work remotely a few days each week
- To always have at least one project that involves design work or content development
- To remain healthy and strong as I get older

How best to support me

- Let me start my work day at 9am. That gives me time for exercise in the morning, which is important to me.
- Email is the best way to reach me. Scheduling a call works too.
- I work best when I know the big picture, so please tell me the purpose of a project, who is involved, the desired outcome, what has been done so far, and then we can explore next steps together.
- I get frustrated when too many details prevent me from having time to be creative and think about big ideas. Let me carve out a chunk of time for a creative project - this is calming and a source of renewal for me
- Give me time to think. I can give you my best work when I've had a chance to "sleep on it."
- Let me know what is working and not working in our work together. I value your contributions and suggestions for improvement.
- Help me maintain work/life balance and my need to feel connected by asking about my family and telling me about yours.

Figure 1.1 Mary Beth's one-page profile

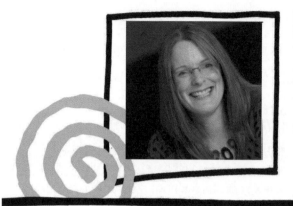

What others like and admire about me

Thoughtful
Inspirational
Passionate about change
Big thinker
Supportive

What is important to me

- To spend time with my family: have an evening or afternoon just with Andy each week; breakfast with everyone together at least three times a week and family night every Sunday.
- To be together with my big extended family for a weekend at least three times a year, and speak to or text my sisters, Nik and Mum every week.
- To work with Julie so that we have great designs and can share what we are learning.
- To spend time with the team six times a year to think together, plan and stay connected.
- To meditate and do a little yoga every day (for 10 -15 minutes) and go to the Saturday class.
- To keep learning new skills. At the moment this is around social media.
- To have a Mac computer, and have my iPhone with me at all times. To keep in touch with people through facebook and twitter.
- Not to work in the evenings or weekends, and only be away from home one night a month for work.
- To be by the sea and walk on Broad Beach as many weekends as I can (usually about 8 a year), and have a family holiday abroad if we can.
- To have hens (currently 3), and cats (3), and spend time pottering in the garden each week.
- To feel that I can make a difference by being part of Circles and in the work that I do with HSA.
- To write to consolidate my thinking, and to share what we are learning. I usually have a writing project on the go.
- To have honest, trusting relationships with everyone who I work with.

How best to support me

- Know that I get frustrated playing telephone tag. Text and emails work best for me, or booking a time for a call.

- Get back to me when you say you will, and meet deadlines we have agreed or let me know if this is not possible (before the deadline is missed!).

- Know that I drown in detail, but love thinking big picture and strategy.

- Be upfront and straight with me – please don't rely on me second guessing you or picking up hint's. I need people to be frank and honest.

- Know that I get frustrated repeating discussions because we can't remember what we agreed the first time we talked about it. Please make sure we always know who is recording actions in meetings or conversations.

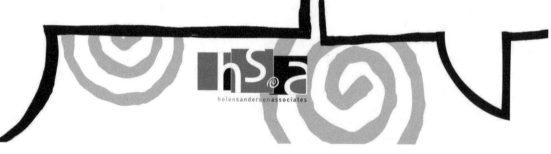

Figure 1.2 Helen's one-page profile

How to support me

- Don't shout at me; if something is important to you, make sure you have my attention, and then tell me.

- If I'm on the phone, let me concentrate.

- Encourage me to go for a run.

Gill was the trainer supporting us in developing one-page profiles. She looked at my one-page profile with me and asked me some thoughtful questions about some of the things that I had stated were important to me. She helped me to transform a one-word statement such as 'running' into a clearer explanation of how far, when and why I wanted to run.

I work in a busy pastoral office between lessons, and Gill also helped me to explain in my one-page profile what I found difficult about working in such a busy and sometimes crowded space. My colleagues then had some clearer ideas about how they could help and understand me. Our pastoral team also took part in some exercises to list each other's attributes, which was a great way for us to bond as a team.

Here is how my one-page profile developed to be more detailed:

Like and admire

Approachable, responsive, organised, engaging.

What is important to me

- Not to be late for lessons.

- To respond promptly to emails and phone calls; to me this means on the same working day that I receive them.

- To have a written record of pastoral decisions made about pupils; this means that I prefer to confirm decisions by email, so that when my memory lets me down, I can remember what was decided and who authorised it.

- It's really important that I eat an evening meal with my family every day, so I should usually leave school by 6pm.

- I am happiest when I run at least ten miles a week – a couple of miles before school every day helps me clear my head and wake up.

How to support me

- Know that not being late for lessons is important to me. Please don't be offended if I have to suddenly end a conversation – I often have to get to the other end of the school site to teach lessons.

- Please read the contents of my emails carefully (I'll try to be succinct) and respond if I have asked for something – I may need this to confirm that we have both agreed to the same plan of action for a pupil.

- If I'm on the phone, let me concentrate.

- Tell me to go home if I'm still at work after 6pm.

Heads of year and other pastoral staff used our own experiences of writing one-page profiles to explain the ethos of personalisation to parents, pupils and form tutors. We showed our early drafts, and also our final one-page profiles, as examples of the process we had been through, to define exactly what was working well for us, and also aspects of our lives that we wanted to develop.

My one-page profile was also shown to pupils in assemblies and tutorials, so that our pupils could see that making a one-page profile should be an enjoyable and fun experience. Our pupils were keen to embrace the idea, and I knew that they were fully engaged in the process, because pupils started asking me if I'd been for a run yet that day when they passed me on the corridor!

Writing a one-page profile has helped me and my colleagues to support each other more effectively in the daily little things, as well as the big things. The most positive aspect for me has been that one of my colleagues now comes into my office and switches the light off if I'm working too late. I'm getting out running much more than I used to, and I feel I have more energy to teach fun, exciting lessons.

Good practice guidance for one-page profiles

One way to enable team members in developing a *good* one-page profile is to have a consensus on what 'good' looks like, and to provide examples of best practice profiles. Figure 1.3 shows good practice guidelines for one-page profiles.

THE BENEFITS OF ONE-PAGE STAFF PROFILES

Our nightmare is that we create an epidemic of 'good paper' that doesn't result in change. 'Good paper' means that although people get excited about developing one-page profiles, they often get filed instead of being implemented. Now we have electronic versions of good paper, which are 'good electronic paper' that keep a record of one-page profiles, but by themselves, this cannot result in creating a person-centred culture.

One senior manager said, 'Staff do have a one-page profile, but they're not sure why they have one or what to do with it next.' Therefore, to avoid a 'good paper/good record' nightmare, a team leader must stay focused on the team's purpose: what are they trying to achieve? And what are the benefits of having a one-page profile?

These same questions were asked by social care provider staff who'd been asked by their managers to develop one-page profiles. They had all come from other organisations where they had experienced a blame culture and were suspicious of why the managers wanted them to develop one-page profiles and how they would be utilised. We were brought in to illustrate eight ways the staff would benefit from writing one-page profiles.

One Page-Profiles
Good Practice Guidance

Photo
Each one-page profile has a current photo of the person

Appreciations

This section is the positive characteristics, qualities and talents that the person has. It can also be called 'like and admire'. It is not a list of accomplishments or awards, it reflects what others values and appreciate about the person.

It needs to have strong, positive statements, and not 'usually' or 'sometimes'

What is important to the person

This is a bullet list of what really matters to the person from their perspective (even if others do not agree). It is detailed and specific. This section needs to have enough detail so that someone who does not know the person can understand who they are. It is not a list of likes and dislikes, it reflects what and who is most important to the person.

The detail is crucial – it should not be a list of one-word bullet points like 'having fun' and instead have the detail explaination of what that means to the person, for example, "I enjoy harmless practical jokes and time to sit and relax with people over lunch or coffee" . It should not include 'regularly' as this means different things to different people, instead, say specifically how often – daily? weekly? monthly?. Rather than saying 'friends' or 'family', write peoples names. It could include:

- Who the important people are in the person's life, and when and how they spend time together.
- Important interests and hobbies, and when, where and how often these take place.
- Possessions that are important to the person
- Information about the rhythm and pace of life, and any important routines.

How to support the person

This is a bullet list of how to support the person, and what people need to either know or do. It is not a list of general hints, it is specific enough that if you were suddenly in a position to support the person, you would know the most important things to do. It can include both what is helpful, and what is not.

Again, the detail is important, so that people would know exactly what good support looks like, rather than a list of short phrases.

Instead of 'stay positive', it is more helpful to explain what that means to the person, for example, "I am a glass half full person and it helps me enormously when people look for solutions and not problems. I find it very draining if I am the only optimist.

Figure 1.3 Good practice guidance for one-page profiles

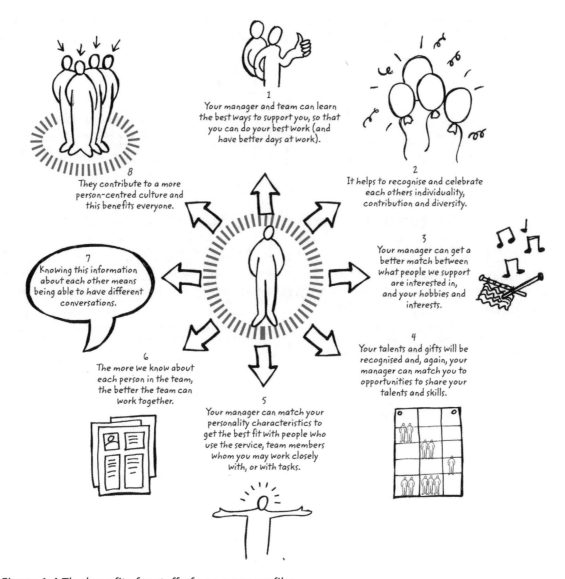

Figure 1.4 The benefits for staff of one-page profiles

Start with introductions

When organisations begin to use one-page profiles they often start by using them for introductions. Rowan joined a new team to help with our communications. At her first team meeting each team member introduced themselves by sharing something from their one-page profile that reflected what was important to them. One-page profiles can also be used as a way to tell people about you outside your team.

Certitude is a leading not for profit provider of person-centred and recovery-focused care and support for people with learning disabilities and mental health needs. The organisation believes that everyone has the right to a good life and uses co-production, community connecting and creative communication to help make this a reality for the 1500 people it supports. Certitude is a merger of two organisations in London. After the merger, the new board of directors developed their one-page profiles to get to know each other better. The directors wanted their website to reflect how far they had travelled to become a person-centred organisation. Typically, information about directors on websites is restricted to a 'designed-to-be-impressive' brief resume. At their team meeting they considered the pros and cons of putting their one-page profiles on the website.

Every member of staff was expected to have a one-page profile, so having the directors' profiles on the website demonstrated that they were 'walking the walk' in this. Other pros were that it showed the directors as people, not just as workers, and also it was a way of staff seeing the quality of profiles that they were looking for. Their concerns, the cons, were that staff, or competitors, could take statements in their one-page profiles out of context or misinterpret them; for example, in the appreciation section of Sanjay, the Finance Director, was the statement 'not a typical FD'. This was a compliment, as Sanjay is warm, personable and focused on ethics and values, and did not fit the dry stereotypes of FDs. He was concerned that the statement 'not a typical FD' could be misinterpreted negatively. Two other directors were worried about the level of detail from their personal lives that they had shared, but Mark, the HR Director's attitude was that his profile reflected who he is, and he was happy to share this.

They decided that the pros outweighed the cons. To avoid the risk of people feeling exposed, each director had two weeks to edit out any statements that they were uncomfortable with. To avoid the risk of misinterpretation, all the one-page profiles were given to a 'critical friend' outside the organisation to see if anything could be misinterpreted that would reflect poorly on the individual or organisation.

If you go to the Certitude website, you can now 'meet' the directors in a very different way, through their one-page profiles (www.certitude.org.uk).

Dimensions is a leading provider of services for people with learning disabilities and people with autism. A not-for-profit organisation, it supports around 3000 people and their families throughout England and Wales, enabling people to live a full life in the community and make their own choices and decisions.

As another example of how to begin with introductions, Sanchi – who works with the Marketing and Communication team at Dimensions – explains how they developed their own profiles to introduce team members:

> Last year we were asked to deliver a 10-minute presentation to a bunch of our colleagues on what the Marketing and Communication team do.
>
> How could we do something creative and original that wouldn't bore everybody rigid, we asked ourselves? How could we convey the complexity of our work and our expertise in ten minutes?
>
> One of our team [members] had the idea of developing a one-page profile for the team. It would serve to introduce us and try to convey what we do, while also sending important messages about how best to work with us so that we can be effective together.
>
> I was tasked with asking internal colleagues what they like and admire about us. I think it is very important in a one-page profile to ask people to contribute and not make that up. Too many people write what they imagine people like and admire about them without actually asking. So we got a good response and that made the team feel proud. The one-page profile turned out to be an ideal opener for a presentation: personal, concise and creative. More and more teams within the organisation have followed suit.

Managers at Dimensions have a link to their one-page profiles as part of their email signature. In this way, everyone to whom they send an email has an opportunity to learn more about the person sending the email. If you go to the head office of another organisation, Real Life Options, you will see the one-page profiles of the directors framed on the walls. Real Life Options is a national voluntary organisation providing specialist care and support. It employs over 1800 people and is involved in the lives of 750 people who have a diagnosis of a learning disability or autism.

Matching staff to people, tasks and roles

For organisations that provide support to individuals, it's vital to get the best match between the individual and the staff or volunteers who provide that support.

The person-centred thinking tool that you can use for this is called 'matching support' and is a way to list the support needed for an individual, and the skills, characteristics and interests that it would be optimum to find in staff or volunteers. Most managers know the skills of their staff, but to be able to make a good match, you also need to have information about characteristics and interests. A detailed one-page profile will provide that information (Figure 1.5).

Bruce Lodge is a care home where 43 people with dementia live. They introduced one-page profiles for volunteers, both to help them get to know the volunteer quickly and how to support them, and to match the volunteer to people who live at Bruce Lodge. They decided to add a section about what volunteers would like to do in the future, so that they could match people according to shared interests.

Performance management

A national organisation that provides support to people with learning disabilities sees one-page profiles as integral to performance management. New staff members and their managers normally start their one-page profile during the induction training.

Three times a year, in their one-to-ones with their manager, they update their one-page profile, if necessary, and talk about whether they are getting the support described in their profile and how they are doing using the person's gifts and talents in the workplace.

At the annual appraisal, both the staff member and the manager write what is working and not working from both of their perspectives and use this as the basis for review and action planning. Another organisation does the same, and is using that information to contribute to its business planning in place of the usual staff satisfaction survey. At the appraisals, when staff have completed their working/not working points and acted on this, the manager asks for the top two working/ not working themes. This information is collected for each staff member and used anonymously to identify the general themes that are working/not working for all staff. The information is then used within the business plan.

From a one-page profile to a person-centred team plan

Once everyone in your team has one-page profiles completed, they can begin a team one-page profile. When the leadership team at Certitude completed their one-page profiles, they spent 40 minutes looking at the common themes and pulling together a first draft one-page team profile (Figure 1.6).

Their one-page team profile had five sections:

- Our purpose

- Great things about us

- What is important to us

- How we support one another

- How others can support us.

Borough Care

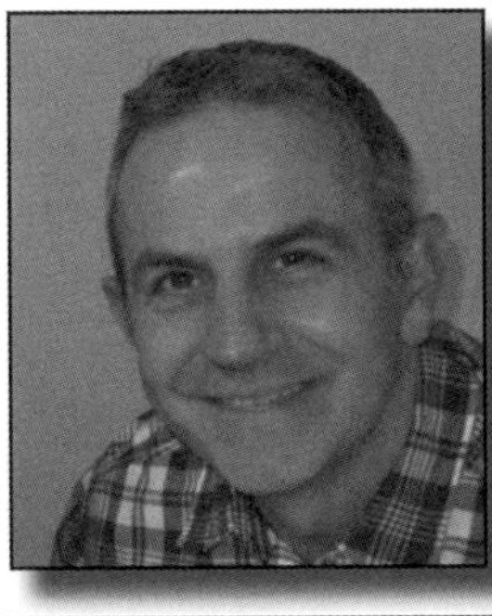

What people appreciate about me
Big foodie and great cook, goes the extra mile to help, patient, caring, conscientious, organised, positive attitude.

What's important to me

- My family, Helen and my three daughters Ellie, Laura and Kate.
- Speaking to my brother every week, and texting a couple of times a week.
- Good freshly ground coffee – everyday
- Good wine – at the weekend.
- Eating out - trying new restaurants when we can.
- To be fit - cycling (weekend cycling with friends) and swimming each week.
- Being organized and prepared.
- Going to the cinema a couple of times a month (anything except rom-coms).
- Having barbecues in the garden when the weather is warm enough.
- Learning Spanish (class on Monday evening).

If I could I would

- Go wine-tasting.
- Train as a barista.
- Go power boating.
- Go outdoor swimming.
- Go canoeing in an Indian canoe (lake not sea).
- Explore Manchester a (art galleries etc.).

How best to support me as a dementia friend

- I need to feel confident that I can support the person that I am matched to, and have all the information I need.
- To arrange in advance when I am going to visit, and have as much notice as possible if things change. I would hate to turn up and things have changed and not be told.
- Contacting me by my mobile is best.
- To know who to contact if there are any problems.
- To be honest and direct with me if things are not working out.

Figure 1.5 One-page profile for a volunteer

For many teams, a one-page team profile is a way to get started in building a person-centred team plan. As you can see in Figure 1.7, you can start with one-page profiles and then add information about purpose, performance, processes and progress to build from one-page to a full plan.

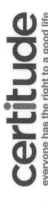

certitude
everyone has the right to a good life

CERTITUDE'S LEADERSHIP TEAM PROFILE

Our Purpose: Working as a team and acting with integrity we will lead the organisation to achieve its vision and mission through listening to and learning from the people we support, our workforce [staff and volunteers] and the external market.

Great things about us

Aisling is reliable, has high standards and stamina
Marianne is creative, motivating and questioning
Mark is dependable, knowledgeable and a good listener
Mary is decisive, steadfast and encouraging

Janette is organised, loyal and committed
Sanjay is patient, knowledgeable with a can do attitude
Nicholas is creative, determined and open to ideas

What is important to us

- To spend time with people we support and staff so we know first hand that what we are doing is what people want
- To have clear, regularly reviewed, goals and plans that achieve positive outcomes for the people we support
- To celebrate individual, team and organisational achievements
- To organise what we are doing, using project and programme management tools – plan it, do it, not over think it
- To be a unified and effective team – debate, disagree and reaching consensus
- To spend time looking outside our organisation – generating new ideas, keep learning and building connections with others
- To encourage creativity in each other
- To evidence success through people's life stories as well as data about quality and performance
- To balance our time between the 'here and now' and visioning the future

How we support one another

- We take time to get to know each other better and use our one page profiles to share what's important to us as colleagues
- We use positive and productive meetings tools in our meetings
- We share stories of success – keeping focussed in meetings on what is working well, while also looking at what's not working
- We share responsibilities and the workload
- We challenge each other – bringing each other back to purpose and vision
- We share new ideas with each other so we can learn together

How others can support us

- Share good news, success and challenges with us
- Read our one page profiles
- Feedback to us on what we do well as a team and what we could do better

Figure 1.6 Certitude's one-page leadership team profile

Copyright © Helen Sanderson and Mary Beth Lepowsky 2014

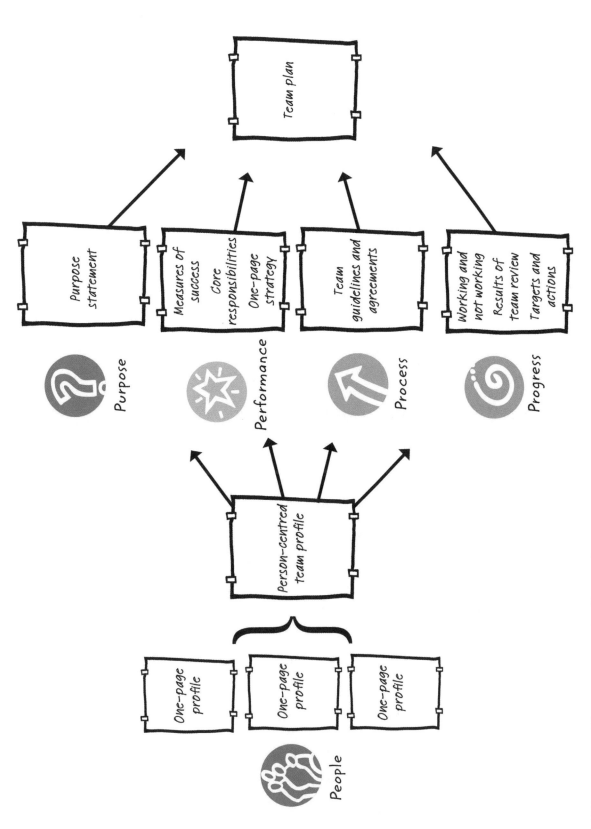

Figure 1.7 One page profile to person-centred team plan

Here are what we see as the benefits of having a person-centred team plan

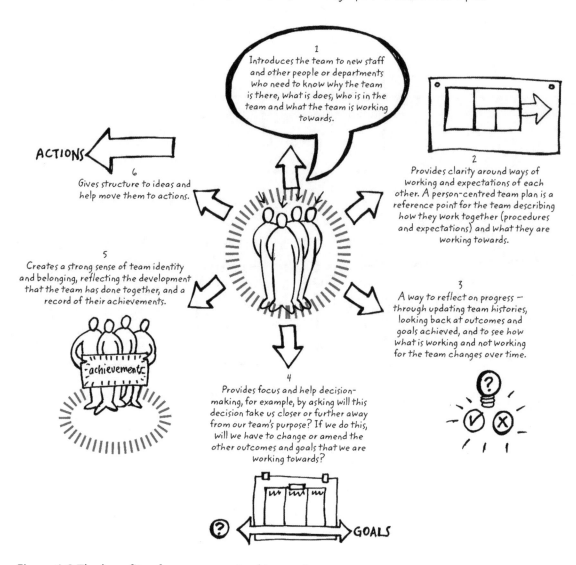

1
Introduces the team to new staff and other people or departments who need to know why the team is there, what is does, who is in the team and what the team is working towards.

ACTIONS

6
Gives structure to ideas and help move them to actions.

2
Provides clarity around ways of working and expectations of each other. A person-centred team plan is a reference point for the team describing how they work together (procedures and expectations) and what they are working towards.

5
Creates a strong sense of team identity and belonging, reflecting the development that the team has done together, and a record of their achievements.

3
A way to reflect on progress – through updating team histories, looking back at outcomes and goals achieved, and to see how what is working and not working for the team changes over time.

4
Provides focus and help decision-making, for example, by asking will this decision take us closer or further away from our team's purpose? If we do this, will we have to change or amend the other outcomes and goals that we are working towards?

GOALS

Figure 1.8 The benefits of a person-centred team plan

Here is what you could expect to see in a person-centred team plan, related to the five Ps in person-centred teams.

Table 1.1 *The five Ps*

Purpose	• A statement of purpose, or graphic.
People	• One-page profiles for each team member, including what people appreciate about them, what is important to them as a team, and how they want to be supported.
Performance	• Usually a one-page strategy about what success looks like and how it can be measured. • Doughnut: What core responsibilities are, and where they can be experimented with in delivering success.
Process	• Team guidelines: How a team works together.
Progress	• What is/isn't working? • Targets and actions to improve.

A person-centred team plan is a compass for the team. It enables team members to see where they are now, and the direction that they are heading in. Figure 1.8 demonstrates what we see as the benefits of having a person-centred team plan.

Throughout the book we will come back to person-centred team plans, and one-page profiles within them. Mike Figliuolo, in his book, *One Piece of Paper*,[6] points to the power of a leader describing their values on one page, through what he calls leadership maxims. One-page profiles reflect the person's values and also share their passions, what matters to them and, importantly, how to support them to be successful. One-page profiles and person-centred team plans are living descriptions of the person and the team; they are added to and updated over time; they are reference points for team decision making, and a record of progress.

A person-centred team plan and the process of becoming a person-centred team starts with purpose, which we introduce in the next chapter.

Chapter 2

Purpose

> I'm doing what I think I was put on this earth to do. And I'm really grateful to have something that I'm passionate about and that I think is profoundly important.
>
> *Marian Wright Edelman (American activist for the rights of children)*[7]

What would your staff members say if they were asked to define your team's purpose? Everything in a person-centred team begins with and returns to purpose. Being part of a team that honours and values what is important to the individual can provide an extraordinary sense of fulfilment. As Marian Edelman suggests in her quote, having a clear vision makes sense in order to live a purposeful life. If personal purpose is not aligned with the team's purpose, the ill fit can impact on the team leader, their colleagues and ultimately the quality of work they all deliver.

In this chapter we share person-centred thinking tools to discover, confirm and develop your team's purpose, different ways to record or communicate this and how this is the start of your person-centred team plan.

Purpose questions

In this chapter you will answer these questions about your team's purpose:

- Why are we here?

- Why am I part of this team?

Here are the person-centred practices that can help you address the questions around your team's purpose.

Table 2.1 Addressing the purpose questions

Purpose question	You will have finished this section when...	Helpful tools
Why are we here?	You're clear about the contribution your team makes to the organisation's mission.	Purpose from different perspectives communicated via a statement, purpose poster or part of a one-page strategy.
	Your team's purpose has been co-created with all members of the team.	Defining impact. Appreciative visioning. Negative brainstorming.

| | Team members can describe the team's purpose in their own words. | 'Front Page News' visualisation to communicate clearly your purpose, or a purpose poster. |
| Why am I part of this team? | You're aware of your own purpose and values, and how they align with team purpose. | Personal values. |

Why does 'purpose' matter?

American businessman and educator, Stephen Covey, told a story about staying in a hotel and being impressed by the exceptional service he received from the staff. He was so impressed that he sought out the manager to ask how he had been able to create such exemplary service. The manager explained that each team had developed a custom-tailored purpose statement connected to the overall mission of the hotel, but expressed it in their own language.

Person-centred teams have a clear, compelling and shared sense of purpose that is closely aligned with the mission of the organisation. Clarity about the common purpose – at both a personal and a team level – that aligns with the organisation's vision, mission and values is more likely to lead to exceptional performance.

A shared sense of purpose means:

- When a team have developed a shared vision and purpose, they can easily agree on what needs to be done to achieve it.

- When people work to create a preferred future they helped to define, they are happier, more motivated and more productive.

- When team members understand the team purpose, they find greater meaning and personal satisfaction in their own contributions.

- Satisfaction contributes to staff retention, which in turn helps the financial bottom line.

President of Momentum LLC, Deirdre Maloney[8] writes that there are two reasons why teams need a purpose:

- Sense of ownership, which moves employees from compliance to commitment.

- Compelling motivation to work hard and strive for continuous improvement.

Earlier we posed the question, 'What would your team say if they were asked to define your team's purpose?' Many teams skip the essential stage of defining their purpose, which makes them less likely to achieve their goals and objectives. Other teams discount the significance of a purpose statement altogether. So it's not uncommon to get a restating of the organisation's mission statement since few people fully comprehend what that means within the context of their team's purpose.

Being clear about purpose influences everything else. It is vital to get this right at the beginning. What if your team never took the time to define its purpose? If it doesn't happen at the onset of a team's formation then you will need to recreate it now. You can turn it into a team-building opportunity that enables team members to reflect on and create their team's purpose, in the context of the organisation's mission, vision and values.

What do we mean by 'purpose'?

Before we proceed any further, we want to clarify our meaning of purpose and how it relates to mission-related terms:

> *Vision:* The desired future state of the organisation; a long-term view of what would be different if the work was completed.

> *Mission:* A statement that describes why the organisation exists and what it does in order to achieve the vision.

> *Values:* Define what matters most to people within the organisation; how it influences how the mission is enacted, and guides decisions and behaviour.

> *Team purpose:* Expresses the contribution a group makes towards fulfilling the organisation's mission.

> *Individual purpose:* A statement that describes what an individual team member is passionate about, and draws them to their chosen line of work.

A team's purpose provides *positive tension* that keeps it striving to fulfil its purpose. Imagine a rubber band that, when stretched, creates a tension that causes the band to return to its desired future state. A team 'stretched' by challenges and opportunities should be able to rely on a compelling purpose statement that helps them to focus and refocus, thereby pulling them back into shape and holding them together.

Who decides on the team's purpose?

Sometimes teams are created to deliver specific objectives. The organisational leadership creates the initial purpose or 'charge' to the team, department or committee. There are times when it's necessary for team leaders to suggest the initial purpose to provide context, but person-centred team members are encouraged to co-create that purpose and explore their own values and aspirations in relation to it.

If team members are not given the opportunity to discuss their individual hopes and dreams for the future, they'll be less likely to contribute to or commit to the organisation's mission. The process of arriving at a shared purpose is as important as the final purpose statement itself. Following are some opportunities and challenges of co-producing a team purpose statement.

Table 2.2 *Opportunities and challenges of co-producing a team purpose statement*

Opportunities	Challenges
Greater innovation.	Less control.
Buy in.	Takes time and can slow the process.
Increased clarity.	Divergent individual perspectives can inform and influence, but shouldn't override what is important for the team as a whole.
Increased commitment.	
Develops relationships.	
Creates alignment.	
People who are affected should have input.	

The act of co-producing the team purpose helps people to buy in and assume ownership of the ensuing work and outcomes. This provides an alignment of individual, team and organisational purpose that will lead to positive results.

People who work collaboratively to define their team purpose are better equipped to negotiate challenges and conflict. The team purpose is a grounding element that should remain constant as it is the foundation for future goals and actions. People can then rely on the purpose statement to refocus the team during confusing or chaotic times.

Who needs to be involved?

It may not always be practical or possible to involve all stakeholders in the development of the team purpose. As a leader you must ask yourself what is the appropriate level of involvement of those who will be affected? Who should be involved? And why and how should they be involved?

If it's not practical for everyone to be present during the decision-making process, perhaps team representatives can be nominated. For example, Rovi – Executive Director of Orcutt Area Seniors in Service, Inc. (OASIS)[9] – did exactly this as she prepared her board of directors to revisit their purpose statement.

Rovi invited Mary Beth to ask the board to consider the question 'Why are we here?' while clarifying their main purpose. Since it wasn't practical for all members of the organisation to participate, Rovi collected input from a survey that asked what was most important when considering programmes, services and leadership roles.

The board used this member input as they reflected on their mission and vision from different perspectives. And from there they drafted a purpose statement:

Our purpose in relation to our members is to:

- provide a facility, programmes and services that meet their needs

- listen to members and keep them informed

- encourage member participation and involvement

- be responsive to the needs of members by approving programmes they want.

Our purpose in relation to each other on the board is to:

- remain open to each other's ideas and opinions
- provide moral support and back-up support of knowledge, ideas and time
- communicate well with one another
- follow policy and ensure due diligence
- encourage and respect one another.

Our purpose in relation to the Luis Oasis Senior Center is to:

- provide a sound, safe environment
- ensure financial stability and fiscal responsibility
- set standards, principles and policies
- provide a security blanket that is a home away from home.

Our purpose in relation to the community is to:

- serve as ambassadors to be the public face of the centre
- provide information, referrals and educational seminars for the community
- educate others about the needs of aging members of the community
- invite involvement from the community
- sponsor other organisations by making our facilities available for use.

Different ways to clarify the team's purpose

Most people acknowledge the importance of having a clear purpose, but many never actually put it into practice. Since no one technique works for every team, the following are some elements you can mix and match to suit your particular situation and culture, which begin with the first of the two purpose questions, 'Why are we here?' and follow with 'Why am I part of this team?'

Purpose question 1: why are we here?
THINK ABOUT PURPOSE FROM DIFFERENT PERSPECTIVES

It's very powerful to think about a team's purpose from a variety of perspectives. Different teams have different stakeholders, and you can think about your team's purpose in relation to each of them. For example, what is the team's purpose in relation to:

- customers or people the organisation supports?
- each other in the team?
- the organisation?
- the community?

For example, a 'supported living' staff team might think about its purpose in relation to the three people with disabilities that they support; an inclusion team may see their primary purpose as enabling staff to work in ways that build community, and therefore the people they support are staff. Similarly, the people that the human resources team supports could include all the staff and managers in the organisation.

Start by thinking with the team about who their stakeholders are, and then decide on the most important ones. Then work together to try to step into the shoes of each stakeholder and reflect on what they want from your team – what they would see the team's purpose as.

A first draft of a purpose statement can be crafted from that information to guide the work and team behaviour until a final draft has been developed. The Luis Oasis Senior Center is an example of how a board team considered their purpose. Here is how a training team, called Housing Associates, started to think about their purpose in relation to their stakeholders – the people who attend their training, the people who commission the training, their team and the organisation overall.

Table 2.3 *Thinking about purpose from different perspectives*

Our purpose in relation to *people who attend our courses*	Our purpose in relation to *people who commission our courses*	Our purpose in relation to *our team*	Our purpose in relation to *the organisation*
To help people develop the skills and knowledge they need to do their job.	To understand the outcomes they want to achieve from the training.	To support each other to deliver the best services to course participants and customers.	To deliver our services within budget in a way that reflects the mission, vision and values of the organisation.
To deliver training in an engaging and creative way that respects staff knowledge.	To design a programme with clear aims and objectives to deliver these outcomes.	To learn together and continually improve the service we offer.	

GETTING TO PURPOSE VIA NEGATIVE BRAINSTORMING

In the movie, *It's a Wonderful Life*, Jimmy Stewart was given an opportunity to see how life would have been if he hadn't existed. Getting the team to think in the same way is another way to obtain a purpose. Here are some questions that could be useful:

- What would be different in the world if we did not exist?

- Who would miss us if we did not exist?

- What would they miss us for? What would be missing in people's (community/ organisation's) lives?

- How could they fill that gap without us?

Asking these questions can provide answers about the team's purpose.

USING APPRECIATIVE VISIONING TO GET TO PURPOSE

The word 'appreciative' means showing gratitude. It also means that which adds value, or appreciates. In this context then, appreciative visioning builds on the foundation of what is good about the team. It gets to purpose via a different route by imagining an ideal future (vision), perhaps using graphics and pictures, and how the team can achieve it.

Ask your staff, 'If you woke up in the morning and the world was exactly how you wanted it to be…'

- What would it be like?

- What would people's lives be like?

- What would they be doing? With whom, when and where?

- What is the contribution they can make to the world?

Capture this vision using words, images and colour, and then ask:

- Which part(s) of this can we make a difference to as a team?

- How can our team move closer to this vision?

- What is the contribution we can make to the world?

- What would we be doing? With whom and to what end?

- How would we be working together to achieve this vision?

Another visualisation tool is *Front Page News*. Ask your team which newspaper's front page they would like to be on in the next three to five years. Then ask them to visualise headlines that describe the difference they made, including three stories that illustrate how the team is successful, quotes from influential people describing the difference the team is making and photos that illustrate this success.

If you have a large team you can split it into smaller groups to develop their own *Front Page News*. Then ask each group to jot down common themes to utilise while drafting the team's purpose.

In Warrington, England, the local authority invited several organisations that provide support to people living with dementia to an event that demonstrated national best practices. They asked the teams to envision what successes would be reported in the *Warrington Guardian* newspaper three years into the future. The teams reflected on their purpose in relation to people living with dementia, as well as contributing to the dementia strategy. See Figure 2.1.

CREATE A PURPOSE POSTER

Another way is to create a *purpose poster* or visual representation of your written purpose. You can create a picture of your purpose to make it more visually compelling. When you describe the picture and what it means to you, you use both the imaginative and logical centres in your brain. The pictures show you how team members want things to be. Ask people to explain their pictures to the group as you listen carefully. Figure 2.2 is a purpose poster from a team in Northern Ireland, from Positive Futures, who support families.

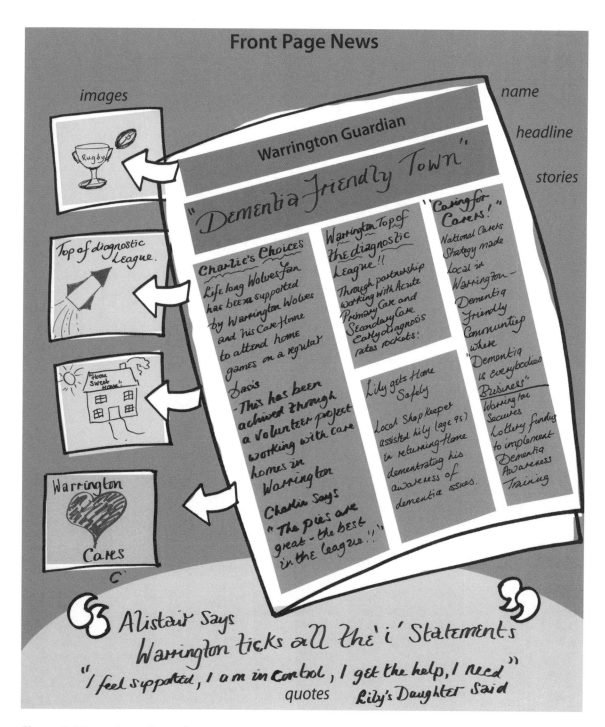

Figure 2.1 Front Page News for Warrington

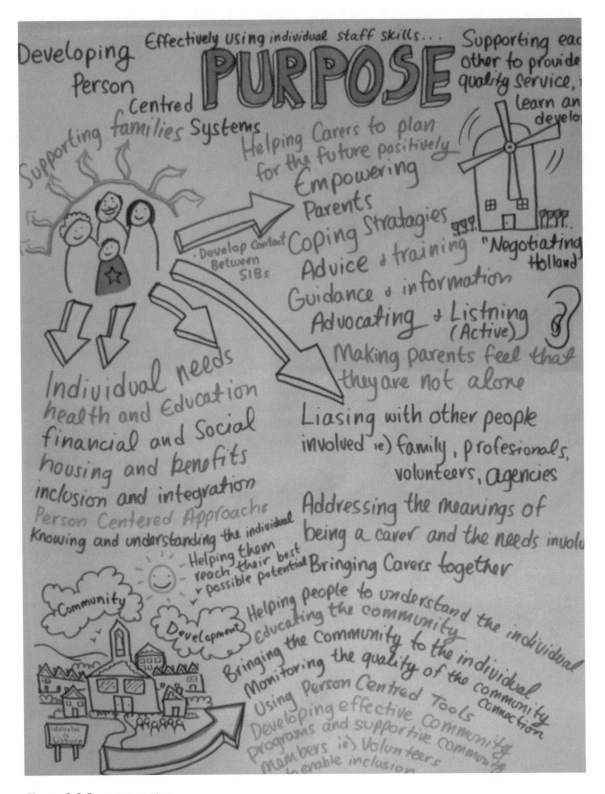

Figure 2.2 Purpose poster

Purpose question 2: why am I part of this team?

Stephen Covey encouraged people to 'begin with the end in mind' (Covey, p.95), meaning, to think about personal purpose and what a life well lived means. Similarly, Jack Canfield – originator of the *Chicken Soup for the Soul* series of stories – encourages his readers to develop personal purpose statements. He shares his own which is: 'My mission on this earth is to inspire and empower people to live their highest vision in a context of love and joy' (www.successwithjack. com/life_purpose.html).

Being passionate about their work connects people to a strong sense of purpose and fulfilment. Co-founder of Apple Computers, Steve Jobs, captured this in his famous quote: 'You've got to find what you love. Your work is going to play a large part of your life and the only way to be truly satisfied is to do what you believe is great work. And the only way to do great work is to love what you do. If you have not found it yet, keep looking. Don't settle' (Stanford Commencement address 2005).

An individual purpose statement answers the question: 'Why am I part of this team?' as it's the framework for creating a powerful life at work, at home and in the community. A strong sense of personal purpose guides people in the decisions they make and in the directions they take.

In the team context, a purpose statement is a guide to all members about who each person is and why the work they do matters.

PRIORITISING VALUES TO CREATE AN INDIVIDUAL PURPOSE STATEMENT

Encourage the team to draft an individual purpose statement by reflecting on their core values. This approach to prioritising values is adapted from Steve Pavlina's writing on personal development, which suggests that an individual purpose statement should answer these three questions:[10]

How would I describe my reason for being (purpose)?

Have your team think about past successes. Identify examples of personal success in recent years – which could be at work, home or in the community – and identify common themes.

What do I stand for (values)?

Ask them to develop a list of values and attributes that identify them and their priorities. Narrow it down to the top ten and then choose five that are the most important (which they can add to their profile to help others understand them better).

What actions do I take to deliver my purpose and my values (contributions)?

Reflecting on the top five values, list ways they could make a difference to the team and organisation. In an ideal situation, how could they contribute best to:

- the people the organisation supports?
- other members of the team?
- the organisation itself?
- the community?

Following is how one educator arrived at her individual purpose statement.

Successes

- Led a team to develop a public charter school.
- Initiated and delivered religious services to families in rural areas where there were none.
- Facilitated numerous non-profit teams to create strategic plans.
- Coached individuals to achieve goals in personal and professional growth.

Themes

- Successes relate to developing a shared vision, building capacity and creating better communities.

Top ten core values

- Family
- Community
- Connection
- Creativity
- Helpfulness
- Hopefulness
- Making a difference
- Professionalism
- Acknowledgement
- Resilience.

Top five most important values

- Family
- Community
- Creativity
- Hopefulness
- Making a difference.

Most important value

- Making a difference.

Contributions

- *The people the organisation supports:* Deliver training to staff and providers that help people achieve what they want in life. To have a lasting impact on the way people live their lives.

- *To other team members:* To be an example in terms of considering multiple perspectives, and offering a compelling vision of what is possible and steps to get there.

- *To the organisation:* To give team leaders and supervisors skills and tools to lead high-performing teams.

- *To the community:* To use my talents in such a way as to strengthen families and communities.

Personal Purpose Statement

- My purpose on this team is to be a catalyst and vehicle for change for the betterment of the community.

ALIGNMENT OF PERSONAL AND TEAM PURPOSE

Helping people understand how their work contributes to the big picture is one of the most important roles of leadership. We believe it's a team leader's core responsibility to ensure that their purpose is clearly defined, clarified and shared. A team leader can use team members' values to create an alignment of individual and team purpose.

Once the team identify their top five values and share their purpose statements, look for common themes then ask them to discuss:

- What values and beliefs guide our daily interactions?

- When we need to make hard decisions, what do we base them on?

- What values and beliefs do we want our team to reward?

- What are we really committed to?

The team can add those values to their plan to fine-tune their purpose statement.

Getting started

We hope that by now you have some ideas about how your team can answer the questions 'Why are we here?' and 'Why am I part of this team?' Creating a clear purpose is essential to delivering team results. It's like a ship's rudder, and you want to make sure the purpose is strong and 'seaworthy' before sailing to a new destination.

Make it clear

Don't assume the benefits of aligning team purpose are as clear to others as they are to you. Be aware that what one person considers to be a benefit might be different to the next person. Give people the opportunity to discuss the benefits and consider 'What's in it for me?'

A good indicator of a clear purpose is when team members can easily describe it to others in their own words. If your team co-created the purpose statement and still can't describe it, then it's not as clear as you may think and will need to be reworked.

Make it relevant

To get maximum buy-in and commitment – and ultimately better team results – the purpose needs to be something everyone wants and is linked to the needs, interests and goals of individual team members within the context of the organisation's mission.

Make it simple and meaningful

The objectives of the team must not only be relevant, but also worth the effort. The organisation and its staff must realise a meaningful outcome as a result of the effort.

Eliminate overused buzzwords and make things easier to comprehend. For example, one team decided their purpose was: 'To ensure that all people served by our organisation have a person-centred plan in place that is updated annually according to their birth month.' This is a crystal clear purpose.

Make it doable

Keep members motivated with a purpose statement that challenges the team to stretch (like the rubber band mentioned previously), and is positive and possible. Everyone wants to be part of a successful team; therefore, if team members believe the purpose can't be fulfilled, they'll likely disengage and become discouraged.

Make it compelling

Create a sense of urgency to drive motivation and team-work. Find ways to communicate why the team needs to become involved as a way of building momentum.

How to record this in your person-centred team plan

Creating the team purpose is a significant step towards understanding all five elements of a person-centred team, and the first step in developing a person-centred team plan.

After the purpose statement is done, keep it visible as a reminder of what the team wants to achieve. Post it in the office, add it to meeting agendas and minutes, and refer back to it when making important decisions. Keep it updated as significant changes within the team or organisation occur.

You'll want to embed the purpose statement into the team plan as a useful tool to guide your team through opportunities, challenges and changes. One way to do this is with a team foundation template – a graphic one-page person-centred team plan.

You can create a person-centred team plan utilising *Word*, *PowerPoint* or other design programmes.

The leadership team of NorthStar Supported Living Services in California used *PowerPoint* to build their team plan. In Figure 2.3 they list their team purpose along with their core values.

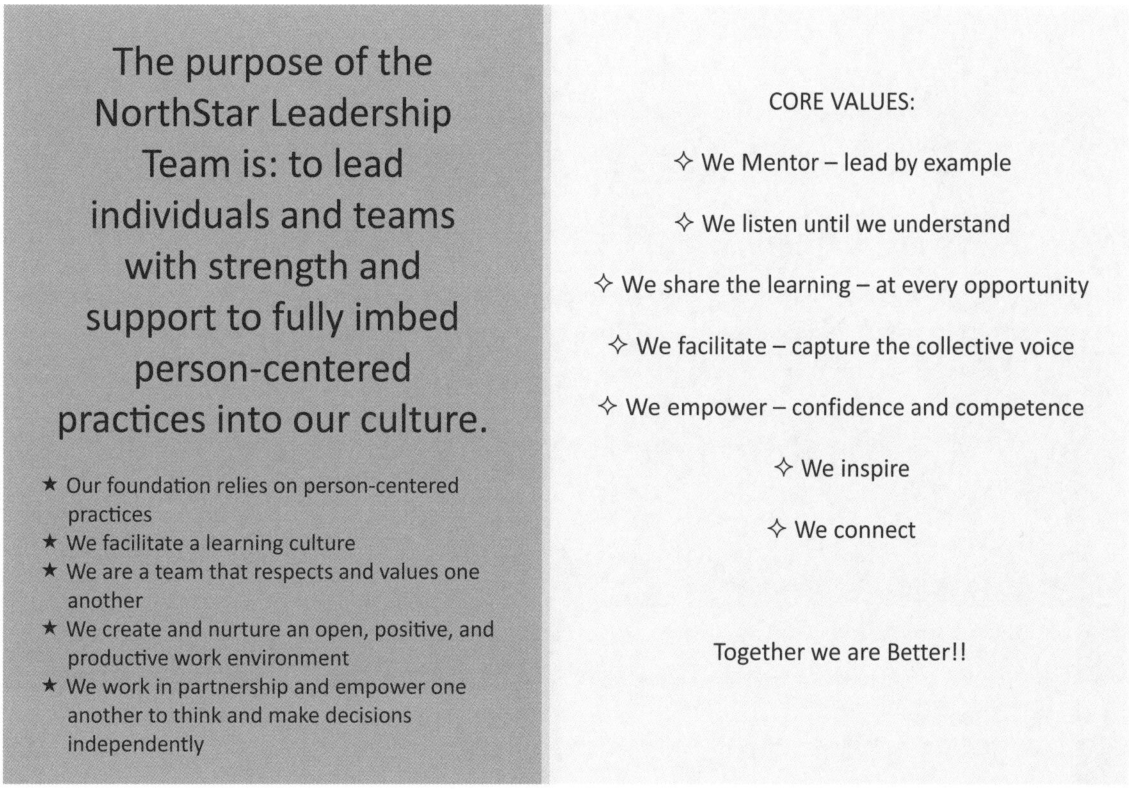

> The purpose of the NorthStar Leadership Team is: to lead individuals and teams with strength and support to fully imbed person-centered practices into our culture.
>
> ★ Our foundation relies on person-centered practices
> ★ We facilitate a learning culture
> ★ We are a team that respects and values one another
> ★ We create and nurture an open, positive, and productive work environment
> ★ We work in partnership and empower one another to think and make decisions independently
>
> CORE VALUES:
>
> ✧ We Mentor – lead by example
>
> ✧ We listen until we understand
>
> ✧ We share the learning – at every opportunity
>
> ✧ We facilitate – capture the collective voice
>
> ✧ We empower – confidence and competence
>
> ✧ We inspire
>
> ✧ We connect
>
> Together we are Better!!

Figure 2.3 The purpose and core values of the NorthStar Supported Living Services in California

The Oxnard Children's Team from Tri-Counties Regional Center in California used free photo templates from www.smilebox.com, and inserted a team photo and images of their purpose statement and core responsibilities created in *PowerPoint* (see Figure 2.4).

A clear purpose is grounded in values and provides a compelling reason for coming to work each day. It's the compass that keeps the team aligned with the organisation's mission by:

- recognising what progress is being made

- determining whether the team is on or off track

- identifying what needs to change when things aren't working.

If a team blocks the development of a meaningful purpose statement, there may be other issues that need to be addressed as there might be symptoms of problems in the areas of people, performance, process and progress. In the remaining chapters in this book, you will learn some tools for addressing some of these issues, but the work to address these distractions early on should be with the intent of revisiting and redefining the team purpose. Investing energy and resources in other aspects of work without clarifying purpose can become a misguided effort, leading to wasted time and expense. Aim to clarify your purpose first, and think about what might get in the way of doing that well.

Now that the purpose statement has been recorded in the team plan, you can use the checklist in Table 2.4 to confirm your understanding of purpose. Then you can explore the talents, contributions and support needs of team members in the People chapter.

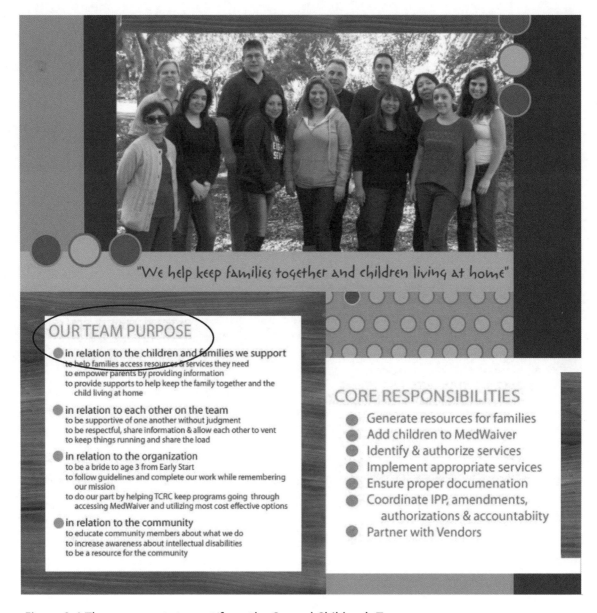

Figure 2.4 The purpose statement from the Oxnard Children's Team

Table 2.4 *Purpose checklist*

Purpose checklist

	Strongly disagree	Disagree	Agree	Strongly agree
I know what contribution our team makes to the organisation's mission.	☐	☐	☐	☐
Our team's purpose has been co-created with team members.	☐	☐	☐	☐
Our team purpose was created after considering perspectives of different stakeholders.	☐	☐	☐	☐
I can easily describe our team purpose in my own words.	☐	☐	☐	☐
I am aware of my individual values and purpose and how they align with the team purpose.	☐	☐	☐	☐
I know how to add our purpose statement/ graphic to our team plan.	☐	☐	☐	☐

Chapter 3

People

> We think of organisations as a network of transactions. They are of course also a social network. Ignoring the people dimension, treating people as simply cogs in the machine, results in the full contribution they can make being lost.
>
> *Will Hutton, Executive Vice Chair of the Work Foundation[11]*

'People are our best asset' is an outdated cliché that represents a half-truth. Jim Collins gets it right in his book *Good to Great*: 'People are not your greatest asset; the right people are!'[12]

Getting the right mix of qualities and characteristics provides a solid foundation for building a strong team. If a team needs to fill a vacancy it's important to recruit a person dedicated to the organisation's mission and team purpose, who shares values aligned with the organisation's values and is compatible with the culture.

The quality of all relationships between team members is a cornerstone to team success. That being said, individual members may have different personalities, techniques and roles, but it's their collective energies that help them to excel. Person-centred teams recognise that their members can be unique and interdependent at the same time.

The previous chapter explored clarifying the overall team purpose. The next task is to understand the people on your team. You need to help team members get to know and support each other well. This understanding will inform decision making, recruitment, team development and action planning.

People questions

In this chapter you'll answer two fundamental questions:

- Who are we?

- How do we support one another?

Professor Jeanne Plas suggests that a person-centred approach to leadership requires a team leader to:[13]

- fully understand and include individual team members' cultural norms and values

- appreciate and support what team members want from their jobs and their lives

- concentrate on one individual at a time.

Person-centred teams accomplish this by using the two people questions above and a variety of person-centred thinking tools to focus on:

- what others appreciate and admire about each person

- what is important to each person now

- what is important to each person in the future

- best ways to support individual team members.

In this chapter are examples of how this information is collected and shared in a one-page profile for each team member, and built into a person-centred team plan.

Table 3.1 shows the person-centred practices that can help you address the questions about the people in your team.

Table 3.1 Addressing the people questions

People question	You will have finished this section when...	Helpful tools
Who are we?	You know what you value and appreciate about each person in the team.	Appreciation.
	You know what's important to each team member about their life and work.	History. Good and bad days (recorded as one-page profiles).
	You know what people aspire to, their hopes and dreams, and what this means in their work life.	Hopes and dreams.
How do we support one another?	You have clear information about what you can do to support each member of the team.	Stress and support.

Why focus on 'people'?

While most people recognise how important it is to have the right people in the team or organisation, recruitment efforts often limit what we know about candidates to skills, knowledge and job-related experience. Teams frequently set goals and develop action plans without knowing the values, contributions, aspirations and needs of individual team members. It's difficult to sustain high levels of achievement over long periods of time if team members don't feel connected to and supported by each other.

The intentional focus of using person-centred tools to understand what matters to people and how to support them well differentiates person-centred teams from more traditional teams. The deliberate focus on people promotes a vibrant team culture where staff are engaged and have greater capacity for working in an emotionally intelligent way.

In the next section we'll look at staff engagement and retention, Emotional Intelligence and the transfer of person-centred ways of working.

Engagement

According to a 2012 study by the Society for Human Resource Management,[14] employee engagement is a top workforce management challenge. Employees become more engaged when they feel positive emotions towards their work, find their work to be meaningful and manageable, and are excited about their future in the company.[15]

The people questions, 'Who are we?' and 'How do we support one another?' build engagement by enabling team members really to know one another and learn how to provide meaningful support to each other. Being supported in this way helps team members to have positive and hopeful feelings about the workplace, even during challenging economic times.

The US Bureau of Labor reports that American workers aged 25–54 spend an average of 8.6 hours a day in work-related activities – more than any other activity, including sleeping and spending time with family.[16] In the UK the Office for National Statistics reports similar findings, with workers spending on average 8.5 hours a day at work.[17] Considering the amount of time people spend at the office and the pervasive challenge of employee engagement, it seems not only sensible but essential to foster a work environment that inspires people to *want* to show up every day. Being engaged is fundamental to quality of life as well as performance. One way to do this is to use the people questions and person-centred practices throughout this book to transform team culture and promote greater engagement.

Gallup, Inc. analysed results of 30 years of polling workers and came up with 12 questions that are part of a Worker Engagement Index[18] (and were popularised in *First, Break All the Rules* by Marcus Buckingham and Curt Coffman).[19]

Within those 12 questions are three that relate to employee engagement:

1. Is there someone at work who encourages my development?

2. In the last seven days have I received recognition or praise for doing good work?

3. Do I have a best friend at work?

We believe that team leaders who use person-centred thinking tools to explore what's important to colleagues and how they want to be supported are more likely to answer yes to these questions.

Person-centred organisations report that paying attention to people in this manner contributes to a positive work environment and better outcomes for employees, as well as those who receive services and team support.[20, 21]

The Gallup findings also showed that having a work environment that promotes positive employee engagement contributes to reduced employee turnover, greater customer satisfaction and employee productivity.[22]

PathPoint, a California-based non-profit organisation offering supported employment and housing support services to more than 2000 people, uses many person-centred practices in staff supervision and team meetings.

Lisa Padgett, Vice President of Operations, reported: 'We were not anticipating this, but our person-centred initiative has resulted in a more positive work culture. We started by incorporating person-centred principles for Positive and Productive Meetings in our management meetings, and it began to trickle down to unit teams and to planning meetings with individuals we support. When we started, our turnover rate of staff was 30 per cent and it is currently 12 per cent. Although economic factors can't be ruled out, we believe this improvement is due in part to the change in our work culture.'

Similarly, United Response in the UK – whose story is described in *Creating Person-Centred Organisations* – saw its staff turnover reduce by 40 per cent after it introduced person-centred practices.

Emotional Intelligence

Person-centred practices support the development of Emotional Intelligence (EI), a set of competencies proven to contribute more to workplace achievement than technical skills, cognitive ability and standard personality traits combined.

Emotional competencies are learned skills that can be developed to achieve outstanding performance. They include social competencies that determine how people handle relationships, and personal competencies that determine how people manage themselves in relationships.[23]

Person-centred practices support core skills that build EI; in particular, competencies of self-awareness, self-assessment and focused listening. Self-awareness and self-assessment are practiced as people analyse their strengths, identify what is most important in their work, and how they want to be supported to perform to their optimum best.

Focused listening is the ability to listen to understand, without distraction or ego. It allows a team leader to step away from their agenda and into another person's shoes. Increased awareness and sensitivity about strengths and needs create an understanding of and respect for everyone's perspectives, and help to incorporate points of view into decision making.[24]

Howard Bousfield, Head Teacher at Norris Bank Primary School in the UK, believes that introducing one-page profiles to his school (to both children and teachers) had a significant difference in this area: 'One-page profiles made a significant difference in enhancing the Emotional Intelligence in the classroom.'

Extending person-centred practices

If your team works in human services of any kind, then employees who experience a person-centred work environment are more likely to become more person-centred in their work with the people they serve.

Channel Islands Social Services (CISS) provides in-home respite care to families in Ventura County, California. The staff are trained in recognising what's important for each person, and record this information in one-page profiles, which they use to gain a better understanding of the needs of employees and the children and families they support.

Edith Wysinger, CISS's Family Services Manager, commented on changes since their team began using person-centred thinking tools, 'We have observed a significant improvement in the stability and satisfaction of caregivers we have matched with families.'[25]

She noted that when team members use the practices to learn about families and staff, parents report that they feel their needs are being considered and met and they appreciate the staff and caregivers' abilities to connect on a more personal level with their children. Also, caregivers experience more satisfaction in their work as a result of being matched with a family that appreciates their skills and personality. Should a change need to be made, both caregivers and families know that person-centred thinking tools can be utilised to find better pairings.

In a person-centred team, members focus on what's important to the individual members now and in the future, as well as what support people need to be in place which enhances engagement, staff retention and Emotional Intelligence.

Know your people

The two questions that we focus on, when thinking about people, are 'Who are we?' and 'How can we support each other?' We can answer these by considering what people like and admire about each other (their gifts and talents), what is important to them now and in the future, and what support they want. This information can be recorded on individual and team profiles.

We now set out some ways to learn about your colleagues using appreciations, histories and a look at what is important in the future, and then explain how to record this information as one-page profiles and as part of your person-centred team plan.

People question 1: who are we?

APPRECIATION

The Oxford Dictionary states that 'appreciation' means recognition and enjoyment of the good qualities of someone or something. When we think about appreciation in teams we look at personality characteristics, values and accomplishments.

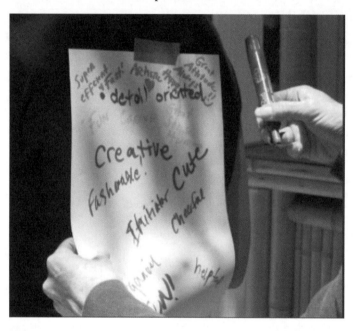

Figure 3.1 Appreciation exercise

There are many different ways to discover what people appreciate about each other, such as:

- During a team meeting, tape a piece of paper to everyone's backs, put some lively music on and ask everyone to walk around writing what they appreciate about each person on the piece of paper. At the end of ten minutes, ask them to share the top three comments they're most proud of.

- Put appreciation cards on a table or the floor and ask people to choose one that says what they appreciate about the person to their right. Then go around the room and ask why they chose them for that person.

- Give members a homework assignment to ask three people in their life (i.e. partner, family and/or friends) for two things they appreciate about them, perhaps writing them on a postcard.

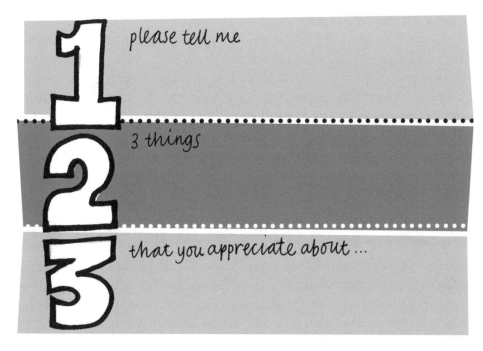

Figure 3.2 Appreciation postcards

Sanchi describes how she approached this with the Communications and Marketing team at Dimensions:

> The whole concept of appreciation and being open and upfront about appreciation is close to my heart. We all tend to ration the positive feedback we give to our colleagues, often without meaning to. We have a staff recognition scheme to reward outstanding contributions, but I wanted to do something a little more personal for my team.
>
> At Christmas I put together a very small set of awards – one for each person in Marketing and Communication. It was a certificate highlighting the positive contribution each person had made in a particular area of their role. Each was a personal reflection on the skills or quality they had demonstrated, alongside the outcomes they had achieved. The presentation was made at our Christmas team meeting, after we had completed the *four-plus-one questions* which we use to review our year and what we had achieved as a team.

However this information is gathered, the next step is to have people choose the top three to five appreciations to add to their one-page profiles. You can also create appreciation books where they can record what people appreciate about them.

In another team, everyone has an appreciation book with their photo on the front. Members are encouraged to record the appreciations they receive through emails, course evaluations or other communications. A couple of times per year everyone brings their book to a meeting and shares one thing they were appreciated for.

Michelle wrote:

> The first time we wrote in each other's appreciation books, I was eager to be able to write down what I liked or admired about the people I worked with. It took me a little thinking time to be able to articulate properly what I wanted to say, as although I knew that I worked with a wonderful, talented bunch of people and enjoyed it when we spent time together, I'd never stopped to consider why I felt this or what specifically each individual brought to the table.

Then, it was time to read what people had written in my book. And even though I knew that I would see messages about what people appreciated about me, I was still delighted to learn what each person felt that I contributed to the team. Some of this confirmed what I knew about myself, such as comments about my 'contagious energy and enthusiasm'. But some were a pleasant surprise, such as, 'your ability to ask questions that help me think better'. This was useful to hear as I also knew that my need to understand things fully, and ask questions until I did, could sometimes be a little frustrating to others.

Having an appreciation book and knowing what others see in me has certainly contributed to me being more self-aware as well as helping me to feel valued by and connected to my colleagues.

LEARNING ABOUT PEOPLE THROUGH HISTORIES

Mary Lou Bourne (owner of consultancy team Support Development Associates) introduced us to a way to learn about someone via their history. She asked Helen to describe seven experiences from her past that made her who she is today (a very powerful way to describe succinctly what has happened in the past) and explain how this influenced what is important to her now.

Jon is a trainer with HSA. One of his all-time favourite positions was as a community nurse. He explained that he appreciated this work as the hours were flexible and he could be creative and use graphics to work with people. He had held a previous position as a manager responsible for 17 staff members: 'That was a dark time for me,' he said, describing the blame culture within the organisation, the inordinate amount of responsibilities he had, the hundreds of emails he had to manage every day and the fact that his manager was always negative about his work.

This immediately gives clues that creativity and being artistic are most admirable traits in Jon, that he prefers flexibility, and that people need to provide positive feedback on his performance.

Another way to learn about people through histories is to capture team history. Mary Beth was working with an adult service co-ordination team in San Luis Obispo, California, that had experienced several years of transition, including a retiring manager, multiple staff promotions and departures, periods of rapid change in legislation, and regulations that affected workloads and services to adults. The team had filled two positions and was preparing to hire one more support staff person.

During a retreat day Mary Beth had the staff created a three-year team history and highlighted the period of rapid change. They first discussed key events and influences, the comings and goings of different people and the emotional impacts the changes had created. They then thought about the aspirations they had at different points throughout those three years (see Figure 3.4).

When they reflected on their history and key insights, they were able to see themes emerging like resilience, positivity, trust, professionalism and peer support. The team members used those insights to update the profile, and at the top of the list was a statement about having time to brainstorm. They discussed how annual retreats had always been, and continued to be, important to allow them to reflect on their relationships and how they work together. The team history affirmed what is important now and would, it is hoped, be so in the future.

They also used what they learned to compile a list of desirable qualities and characteristics to share with the manager responsible for hiring new staff members. All the information collected during the retreat was incorporated into wall posters using sticky notes, which was transferred to a computer document and added to the team plan.

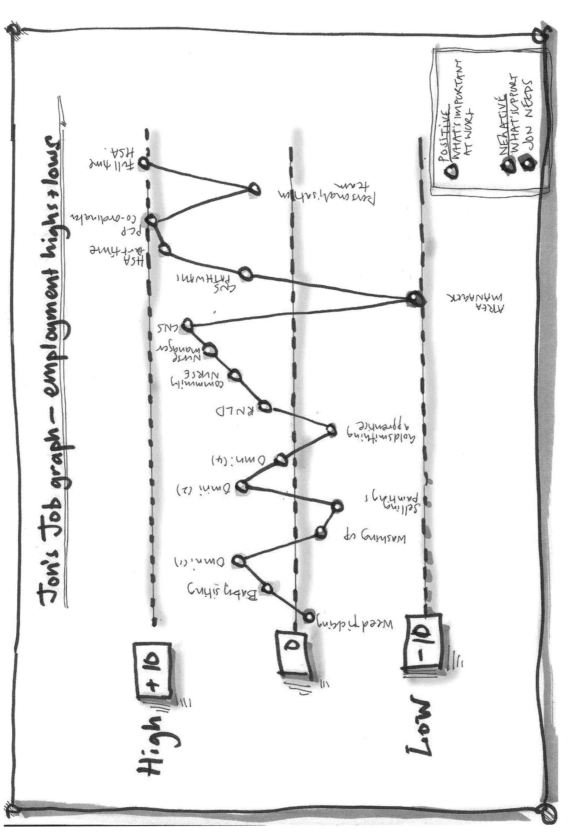

Figure 3.3 Jon's work history

Copyright © Helen Sanderson and Mary Beth Lepowsky 2014

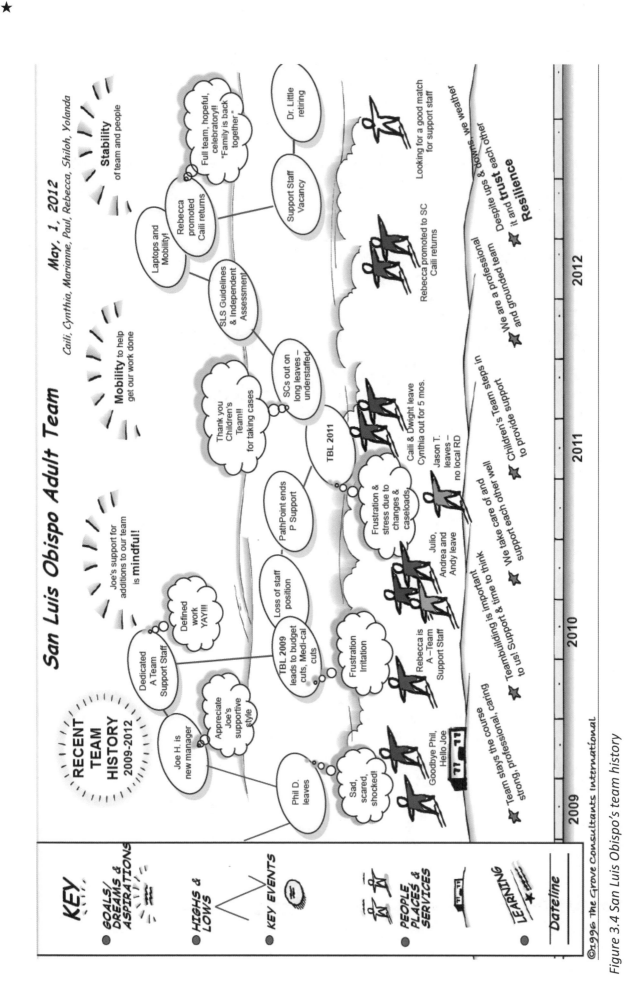

Figure 3.4 San Luis Obispo's team history

WHAT'S IMPORTANT IN THE FUTURE

As well as knowing what's important to people in the present, it's important to learn what they aspire to for the future, such as their hopes and dreams, and what this means in their work life. You can simply ask people where they want to be in a year, but there is another approach. Ask them to imagine that they've awakened from a deep sleep and realise that everything is exactly the way that they would like it to be. Where do they work? What is their role now? Whom do they work with? What is different about their position? Then talk about what this tells you about their hopes for the future.

Motivational speaker, Brian Tracy, says that people can learn a lot about what is important to someone by asking them, in 30 seconds, what their three top life goals are. Knowing what people want for the future can help with making decisions about what opportunities the person could take on within their role now, within the context of the purpose of the team.

People question 2: how do we support one another?

As well as knowing what is important now and in the future, we also need to know how to support and help each other. Person-centred thinking tools like *good days and bad days*, as well as other established instruments can help here.

GOOD DAYS AND BAD DAYS

The tool *good days and bad days* reveals things that matter and is therefore a great starting point to get to know the team from a different perspective. Asking team members what good and bad days at work are like can reveal a great deal about what matters to them and what can help them perform at their best.

You can add this information to their one-page profiles during one-to-one or team meetings and agree on what actions to take to have more good days and fewer bad ones (within the context of the purpose of the team as a whole).

Tim, a manager with Positive Futures in Northern Ireland, reflected on his good and bad days. To him a good day means:

- A cup of coffee just the way I like it!

- I have time to do my work and time to think.

- I have time for my staff.

- I am in touch with what is happening and how my staff are faring.

- I am organised, prepared and in control of my day.

A bad day means:

- Too many meetings, such that I begin to lose focus.

- Going into a meeting knowing there are items on the agenda that I am not prepared for or tasks I have not done.

- I set aside time to do something important but it is hijacked.

From that assessment he ascertained what he thought were the best ways he could be supported, which would mean fewer bad days at work.

To support me really well at work:

- I like being busy, but it is easy to get too busy in this job if you are booking meetings for me. Please check how many I already have on. My online diary is usually up to date. More than three and I start to sink! If you need to put in one over the three, please contact me first and I will do my best to fit it in.

- I want to be accessible to folk who need to talk to me, but there are times when I need space to get on with something. If I need space I will put up a 'Do not disturb' sign. Please try to respect it unless there is something urgent. If there is no sign, I am happy for you to call in. If I can't talk then I will arrange a time to get together.

- Please join me for coffee when you can. One way I like to keep in touch with staff is over coffee/tea in the morning. I also think it helps team relationships for us all to relax and unwind together for a short while. If you are about at coffee time, please come and join me.

- I know that I am not a naturally organised person. I also hate going into meetings unprepared. I am really trying to work on this (and struggling!). If I need to read something in advance of a meeting, please make sure I have it at least three days before. Feel free to check that I have read it.

- I love real coffee – it definitely makes a good day for me! At least two-and-a-half spoons of sugar, and milk. If there is enough hot water, heat the mug first before pouring as it keeps the coffee hot. (I know that I am sad!) More than two cups a day and I will not sleep that night so don't tempt me beyond my capacity. If I am not having real coffee, I will usually take tea.

Another approach is to do this with the entire team to enable them to have more good than bad days, which can lead to:

- information for everyone's one-page profile

- individual and team actions to increase the number of good days people are likely to experience, and therefore improve team well-being within the context of delivering the team's purpose

- development of a set of team agreements about how they work together, and the beginning of a one-page team profile.

The Santa Barbara California Children's Team at Tri-Counties Regional Center used this approach to develop the people section of their team plan. After reflecting on what brings them joy during good days, they created one-page profiles with team colleagues. Then they added them and a section on guidelines to the team plan to help the team have more good days.

STRESS AND SUPPORT

The notion of *stress and support* builds on *good and bad days,* identifies stressors that team members experience, then analyses how they can help themselves and what they need from others. In her blog[26], Helen describes how she started to think about stress and support in her life:

I am passionate about my work and love my family. Sometimes my life gets out of balance trying to juggle both and find time for myself. Does this sound familiar? How do you know when your life is out of balance? What can you do? I want to show how person-centred thinking can help – both on a personal level and also within teams.

Last November, we had a great time workwise – we held two events that were both fully booked and launched two new books, including one at the National Children's and Adults Services Conference in London.

At the same time, I felt my 'balance' slip. It was the 'little things' that gave it away for me. I was catching late trains home from London, grabbing a bag of crisps and perhaps chocolate as I carried on with emails. I noticed that I wasn't sleeping as well, drinking a glass or two of wine every night and skipping my exercise or yoga. My iPhone became an extension of my body and I lost count of the time I looked at my most recent obsession, Twitter.

In the support planning process there is a great question at the end: 'How will we know that we need to review this support plan?' In our personal lives, another way of asking that question is: 'How will we know that things are not going well for us?' The things I have just described are my way of knowing the answer to that question.

I want to get sharper at noticing when I start to get out of balance so that I can do something about it before it gets too bad. It's a bit like the Johari window for me. The Johari window is a technique created by Joseph Luft and Harrington Ingham in 1955 in the United States, used to help people better understand their relationship with self and others. It is used primarily in self-help groups and corporate settings as a heuristic exercise.[27] There are things that I notice that others may not (the extra junk food and Twitter obsession) and then there are things that others notice that I may not be aware of. For example, my husband Andy notices that I am irritable and I don't do my strange 'opera' singing around the house. I wondered what the other people in the office or team notice about me when I am feeling more stressed? What would I want the team to do if they did notice?

In my journal this week, I used the following questions to help me think about this and what I wanted to do about it:

• How do I know when I am feeling out of balance or stressed?

• What do I notice?

• What might others notice?

• What gives me energy or makes me feel good?

• What drains my energy or makes me feel out of balance?

• What can I change this week?

My action plan for getting more balance this week is to make sure I am doing some exercise three times this week; not looking at Twitter after 5pm; taking ten minutes in between meetings to breathe; going to the cinema with a friend and doing the photobook I have been meaning to do for weeks.

It made me think about whether we know this information about our colleagues. In teams that are striving to be 'person-centred' and in families supporting each other, this is important information. How can we tell by people's behaviour when things are tough for them? What can we support them to do for themselves and what can we do to help?

Here is an example of *stress and support* for Vicky, whose manager changed, and the new manager, Michelle, used *stress and support* as a way to get to know Vicky better and learn how she could support her well.

> Vicky had been previously managed by Charlotte who she knew really well and had a great relationship with. When she started to be supported in her role by Michelle, her new manager, they both decided to get to know each other better by exploring what best support looked like. They used the *stress and support* tool to identify how Vicky communicated when she felt things were getting on top of her. Rather than filling in a form, they had conversations that explored times when Vicky had felt under stress at work. They then looked at how this manifested in different situations – at home Vicky might come across as tetchy, but would never show this at work. Once they had determined how Vicky communicated stress and Michelle had spotted things that Vicky hadn't thought of, they identified how Vicky could be more self-aware and how she could have more confidence/control over the situations that arose. They then agreed what Michelle and the team could do to support Vicky in a way that made sense to her.

USING ESTABLISHED INSTRUMENTS

Instruments such as the Myers-Briggs Type Indicator (MBTI), Strength Deployment Inventory (SDI), DISC Personal Profile System and Leadership Profile Inventory (LPI) are a few leadership and organisational development tools that assess individual style preferences, strengths and potential areas for development.

Mary Beth asked the executives and directors at Tri-Counties Regional Center in Santa Barbara, California, to complete the MBTI (one of the world's most widely used personality inventory tools designed to describe how people perceive the world and make decisions)[28] and share their results during a day of team-building and annual planning.

Each director reflected on the information in the MBTI report to create one-page profiles after seeing ways people with different preferences communicate, interact, make decisions and cope with stress during times of rapid change. They were asked to add three to five points under each of the following headings:

- When am I most myself?

- What do others like and admire about me?

- What is important to me in my work with the directors?

- What aspects of my work are most satisfying and energising?

- What provokes stress?

- How can I be best supported in my work with the directors?

The information was recorded in the team plan, added to individual profiles and is now reviewed periodically as a reminder of how to maintain an effective working relationship within the team.

Stephen Stirk, a certified Myers-Briggs practitioner, worked with Helen to develop one-page profiles for each of the MBTI types, and has used these with individuals who know their type as a way to review or further develop their own profile. Helen is an INTJ (introversion, intuition, thinking, judgement), and the one-page profile for an INTJ helped her update and develop her one-page profile (see Figure 3.6).

Vicky Stress and Support			
		What helps	
What makes me most stressed	How do I usually react to being stressed	What I can do	What I would like you to do
When I have too much to do and can't do things properly, spread too thinly. When I haven't got a clear understanding or plan for work that needs to be done.	I panic and think that I can't do it. I get frustrated with myself, resulting in not being able to sleep, this then makes me tearful. I become less tolerant and irritable. I will panic and bury myself away to try to figure out what I need to do, or I will find excuses not to do the work because I can't face it.	Think logically and plan my work realistically. Use my time more efficiently. Explain to others how I'm feeling and ask not to be disturbed whilst working. Use my online diary and reminder sheets to record what I need to do by when. To do lists work well for me. Make sure that I have clarity about what the work entails before agreeing to do it. Ask for clarity from the person who has asked me to do the work.	Understand that if I ask for more time to complete something it is because I am busy. Make sure that I'm not disturbed when I ask not to be, make sure I get to bed early. Ask me if there is anything you can do to help. When I am less stressed, suggest that I go for a walk or play a game to help me to relax. Remember that I am a detail person and that I need to have as much information about the work as possible. Be patient with me and check back with me that I understand what needs to be done. Agree deadlines with me that are realistic.

Figure 3.5 Vicky's stress and support

Generic One Page Profile for INTJ

What People Appreciate About Me

- That I am good at interpreting the facts to come up with insights and possibilities and so contribute original ideas to a team.
- A strong drive to help get things done when I believe in an idea.
- Strong sense of vision and am always looking for new directions and areas to explore.

What Is Important To Me

- To work in a field that appeals to me and be able to reflect in depth about it.
- To be able to be independent and not always forced to conform.
- My work must be completed to a high standard, or I am not satisfied with it.
- To be organised and be able to carry jobs through to the finish.
- Structure and schedules for me to feel a job will be done properly.
- Space for me to develop my own strong ideas of how things should be done, or how life should go.
- To have the facts and ideas behind my work, so I need to draw them out and understand them.
- To work with new complex ideas and to be changing and improving rather than sticking with the status quo.

How You Can Best Support Me/Work With Me

- Present me with the big picture first before we go down into detail, and leave space for me to be creative, and to intellectualise about ideas.
- In meetings, I may be quiet while I am reflecting and thinking ideas through, so you may need to draw me out by asking questions.
- If you want to communicate something important to me, it is better in writing than face to face, email or voicemail.
- Make sure any work you are doing with me or for me is of a high standard.
- If I am sceptical or critical of an idea, please bear with me and talk it through, but let me know if I am being unyielding or unapproachable.
- Understand that my determination to get the job done may feel overbearing to you., but let me know if I am not letting go of impractical ideas.
- When we are working together, let me make a plan and get the workload organised in detail.

Figure 3.6 A one-page profile for an INTJ

PERSON-CENTRED TEAM REVIEWS

We explain how teams can use person-centred reviews in the Progress chapter. While they're typically used to record progress, they can also be used to develop the first draft of a person-centred team plan and capture it in the context of the team's purpose:

- What we like and admire about each other and the team as a whole.
- What is important to us at this point in time.
- What is important in the future.
- How best to support our team.
- What is working/not working from different perspectives.
- Questions to answer and unresolved issues.

Getting started

Knowing about each other, having this information clearly recorded in a one-page profile and incorporating this into a team plan are important aspects in ensuring that you are using everyone's strengths, gifts and talents to deliver the team's purpose, and that each person is supported to do their best work. Here are some considerations as you get started with your team.

MAKE TIME

Dedicate time for individual one-to-one sessions with team members or the team as a whole in a team meeting or time away from the office.

START WHERE PEOPLE ARE

If your team has been working together for a few years and members know each other reasonably well, your first task may be to capture what they already know, then expounding on it with appreciations and histories.

If your team is experiencing difficulties or conflicts, you might want to look at their good and bad days to make sure issues are aired which will lead to productive action. If your team is relatively new, starting with individual histories is a great way to get to know people and to craft their profiles.

LEAD BY EXAMPLE

The most powerful way to enable people to understand the benefits of knowing each other well is to share your own profile.

> Tracey Bush is the Managing Director of Spiral Health and she wanted to introduce one-page profiles to her team of nurses, physiotherapists and occupational therapist in the hospital. She started by developing her own one-page profile and asked a trainer to check it and give her feedback. She shared this with her team to start the conversation about one-page profiles and how they could be useful.

BE CLEAR ABOUT PURPOSE AND QUALITY

Give careful consideration to the quality of the information. Some organisations find it helpful to have a guide that explains why and how profiles are being used, what each of the headings mean and the depth of information required.

> A national organisation in the UK decided it was going to introduce one-page profiles for all staff after piloting this within one of its regions. In the pilot it learned that the staff were suspicious about how the profiles were going to be used by their manager, Julia. Julia's team were worried that they could be moved across teams based on their profiles to get the best 'fit', and that the profiles would be used negatively against them during performance reviews. As a consequence, they wrote profiles containing scant, uninformative details. To address their concerns, Julia created a brief statement about why she wanted staff to develop their profiles, how they were going to be used/not used within the organisation and the required standards of detail (this included some of the benefits to staff described in Chapter 1). This made a big difference to her team's confidence to the point that one-page profiles are now used by the organisation to explain the benefits to others.

DECIDE ON STANDARDISATION VERSUS CREATIVITY

One of the decisions to make early on is whether to have a standardised template for you and your team's profiles or to encourage creativity in profile design.

> Helen was working with a leadership team and this included supporting them to develop their own one-page profiles. She shared with them a range of different one-page profiles done by people in similar organisations. They were initially negative about the standardised template that one organisation had used, and decided that they wanted their leadership team to be able to reflect their personality through their one-page profiles. Helen then used different exercises to enable people to start thinking about what was important to them and how they wanted to be supported in the team. They agreed to bring their first attempt at a one-page profile to their next meeting in a month's time. When they came back together again, people shared their profiles, which had a range of different shaped boxes with clip art and photos. The group talked about their experience of developing and recording their profiles. What emerged was that people had spent more time wondering how to 'design' or illustrate their one-page profile, than they had on the content of the information. Lucy had put what was important to her in a zigzag box, which meant there was only room for three bullet points of information. Julius had more clip art than content. From this, the leadership team decided that they would like to have four different designed formats for their one-page profiles that used their organisation's brand colours and were designed in such a way that there was maximum space for information (which is, of course, the purpose of a one-page profile – to share information). Taking this approach meant that people could choose from one of four designs and could then focus on the information that they wanted to share, rather than the design.

Recording the information in profiles

The processes and exercises introduced in this section lead to both information and actions that can be recorded and shared in three ways:

- Individual one-page profiles.
- One-page person-centred team profile.
- Starting a person-centred team plan from a one-page team profile.

When each person has a one-page profile, this information can be condensed into a one-page team profile that includes the purpose and function of the team, what people appreciate about the team and its members, what is important to the team, and how to support the team to deliver at their best. This team profile can then be modified over time and grown into a more comprehensive team plan that includes more information about core responsibilities, goals and action steps.

By now you will have your statement of purpose. You can begin your person-centred team plan in different ways. Here are a few.

START WITH A ONE-PAGE TEAM PROFILE

Ask each team member to choose two or three appreciations from their one-page profile to go into the one-page team plan. Then look at what is important to each team member – you can create a 'gallery walk' with the one-page profiles on a wall, and then work with the team to pull out themes that are common to the whole team. These can go in the 'What is important to our team' section of your one-page team profile.

Do the same with the 'How to support me' section – share each other's and pull together the common themes. You will now have your first draft one-page team plan. You can also add your purpose statement to it, or have your purpose poster image to go with the one-page team profile. You can see Certitude's leadership team's one-page team profile in Chapter 1 (see Figure 1.6).

USE THE TEAM FOUNDATION GRAPHIC

The purpose will be recorded in the centre of the graphic. Now add each member's information from their profile into the 'What is important to me' and 'How to support me' sections.[29] The Oxnard Children's Team developed their profiles, shared the information as a group, then populated this team foundation with input from each team member.

ADD EVERYONE'S PROFILE TO THE PURPOSE STATEMENT

This will be the beginnings of the person-centred team plan.

SYNTHESISE THE INFORMATION FROM THE PROFILES AND SEARCH FOR COMMON THEMES

Another way to get started is to synthesise the information from the one-page profiles, by looking at what this information says collectively about people. For example, the Oxnard Children's Team considered the information on their team foundation graphic and looked for themes that were important to all team members. They noted those themes in their team plan under sections called 'What's important to us' and 'How to best support us' (see Figure 3.8).

Jim Collins in his book *Good to Great*, stresses that you must *first* get the right people on the bus and the wrong people off the bus *before* you figure out where to drive it. 'First who, then what' is an imperative principle for becoming a great organisation.

His point is that 'who' questions need to come before 'what' decisions, strategy, organisation structure and tactics. When applied to the person-centred team model this means people before performance, before process and before progress.[30]

The team leader should focus on the two people questions and develop profiles to build the team's living record and how each member wants to be supported. With that foundation in place, the work relating to performance expectations, processes of conducting business together and checking on progress will be within the context of meaningful support, which ultimately is the cornerstone of a strong person-centred team.

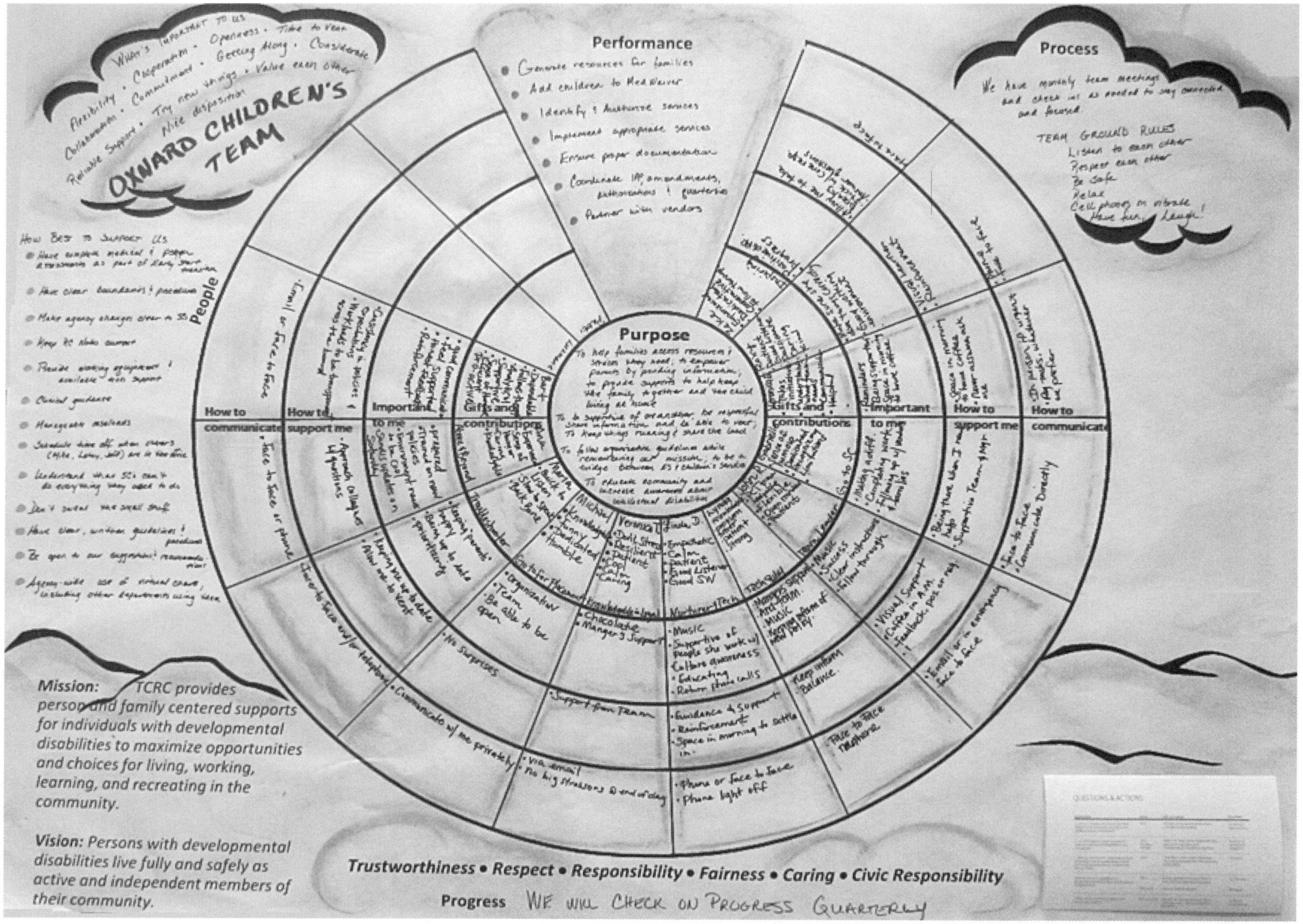

Figure 3.7 Example of a completed team foundation poster

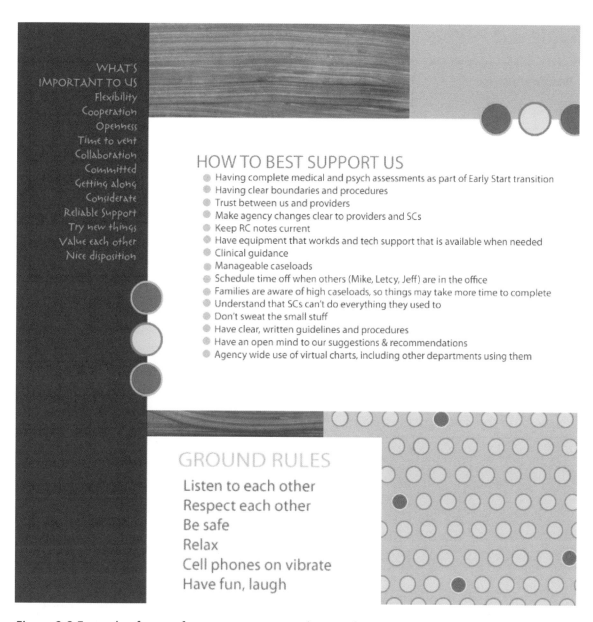

WHAT'S IMPORTANT TO US
Flexibility
Cooperation
Openness
Time to vent
Collaboration
Committed
Getting along
Considerate
Reliable Support
Try new things
Value each other
Nice disposition

HOW TO BEST SUPPORT US
- Having complete medical and psych assessments as part of Early Start transition
- Having clear boundaries and procedures
- Trust between us and providers
- Make agency changes clear to providers and SCs
- Keep RC notes current
- Have equipment that workds and tech support that is available when needed
- Clinical guidance
- Manageable caseloads
- Schedule time off when others (Mike, Letcy, Jeff) are in the office
- Families are aware of high caseloads, so things may take more time to complete
- Understand that SCs can't do everything they used to
- Don't sweat the small stuff
- Have clear, written guidelines and procedures
- Have an open mind to our suggestions & recommendations
- Agency wide use of virtual charts, including other departments using them

GROUND RULES
Listen to each other
Respect each other
Be safe
Relax
Cell phones on vibrate
Have fun, laugh

Figure 3.8 Example of pages from a person-centred team plan

Table 3.2 *People checklist*

People checklist	Strongly disagree	Disagree	Agree	Strongly agree
I know what I value and appreciate about each person in the team.	☐	☐	☐	☐
I know what team members appreciate about me.	☐	☐	☐	☐
I have shared and know what matters to each person in their team, and what their hobbies and interests are outside work.	☐	☐	☐	☐
I am clear about what I need to know or do to support others in the team to work at their best. In turn, my team members know this about me.	☐	☐	☐	☐
I know what my team members want to achieve in the future and they know what I aspire to.	☐	☐	☐	☐
I know how to complete a one-page profile and record this information in a team plan.	☐	☐	☐	☐

Chapter 4

Performance

Focusing on your mission means you are doing good. It does not mean you are doing good well.

Deirdre Maloney[31]

We think that the importance of performance is often underestimated in public sector and non-profit organisations. Indeed, the earlier development of the person-centred team model did not include 'performance' since it was introduced by Mary Beth just a few years ago.

When the team purpose relates to providing support to individuals in health, education or social care, team members sometimes resist defining their performance in clear and measurable ways as they feel the practices are too impersonal, too 'businesslike', and distract from the mission of providing quality services and support.

On the contrary, defining performance helps the team focus on getting results that can lead to significant social change in the most effective and efficient manner. In quality terms this section relates to standards, measures and milestones. Once performance is clear, the team is better equipped to deliver its purpose.

Performance questions

In this chapter we look at what success would look like if your team is achieving its purpose, and how your team can know how well it is doing.

- What does success look like?

- How can we know how well we are doing?

Once performance standards are clear, and your team knows how these will be measured, the next part of the process is how to deliver these. 'Performance' is about expectations and how well you will deliver this; 'Process' is about delivery.

Table 4.1 shows the person-centred practices that can help you address the questions around the performance of your team.

Table 4.1 Addressing the performance questions

Performance question	You'll have finished this section when...	Helpful tools
What does success look like?	You have succinct, shared expectations of what success looks like in practice.	One-page strategy. Starbursting.
	Team members know what is expected of them, and what their core responsibilities are.	Expectation arrow. Doughnut. Competency continuum.
How can we know how well we are doing?	You know how to measure success.	One-page strategy.

Why is performance important?

By now your person-centred team plan should include a purpose statement and useful information about what is important to team members and their support needs. However, as Deirdre Maloney suggests, that alone will not result in positive change and effective work. Teams must go further than focusing just on mission, purpose and people.

Teams need to know what *good looks like* to ensure that people know what their job is, why it's important and what impact it has on others. People can only achieve a high level of job satisfaction when they measure their job performance against a pre-determined standard. If they can't define and measure performance, they'll never know if they have achieved real success. A major cause of stress to employees is not knowing what is expected of them by management and their peers.

Lack of clarity about expected performance and how it will be measured can lead to confusion, frustration and duplication of effort within teams, departments and organisations. With rising competition for limited resources and a responsibility to use public and private capital responsibly, it's important to develop a description of a job done well.

Brian Tracy describes this as a team's *key results area*. He asks the question, 'Why are you paid your salary?' as an indicator of what's expected of the employees and what they are paid to do. He compares these areas to bodily functions: if the body ceases to function it can wither and die. This suggests that without delivering a good performance the team may no longer serve a purpose and its members might lose their jobs.

What is meant by 'performance'?

To deliver high quality services, team members must have a thorough understanding of whom they serve, what they deliver, how well they're expected to do the work (performance standards) and how this will be measured. In order to actualise those standards, they need to understand what is expected from their performance before agreeing to processes and setting goals for improvement (progress).

Aligning purpose, people and performance

In this example, Carolynn, the team leader and her team needed to clarify what their purpose was, and what it meant for their performance. They first started with the organisation's overall mission, what it meant in relation to the employees they support and what they want for their lives, and how to position the team's purpose and performance.

The team supported Anne-Marie and five other individuals who lived together in Old Street in the UK. Before they started working on their purpose and performance, the team saw their role as 'looking after' people and 'taking them out'.

The team were supported to learn about Anne-Marie (and the other people she lives with) in a new way and to look at their role and performance through fresh eyes. With Anne-Marie and her family, and supported by a facilitator, they worked on how Anne-Marie wanted her life to look in a year's time (her outcomes) and what she wanted her life to be like week by week (her perfect week).

When the team thought about the questions 'What support and services do we offer to fulfil our purpose?' and 'How will we know we have been successful?' the answers had to include:

Purpose

- Supporting Anne-Marie in what is important to her in a way she wants to be supported.

Success looked like

- Supporting Anne-Marie to make her own decisions as described in the decision-making agreement.

- Working with her to achieve the actions developed in her person-centred plan and review.

- Supporting her in getting a job.

- Supporting her in her day-to-day life as described in her person-centred plan.

How did they know they were successful?

- Delivering Anne-Marie's perfect week with whatever changes she wanted to make week by week, and analysing her current weeks against her perfect week. Carolynn and Anne-Marie were to review this together each month.

- Anne-Marie's life would be supported to achieve the outcomes from her person-centred plan. They knew this by reviewing her outcomes with her during her person-centred review.

- Anne-Marie would increase the number and range of decisions she made, which were to be recorded on her decision-making agreement and updated every six months.

- Anne-Marie was to include more people in her relationship circle, which would be reviewed every six months.

- Anne-Marie would earn money from a job she enjoyed.

The results presented a significant change in team culture. In the past, the only clear expectations on performance were around financial procedures and recording. Now they were clear about what was expected of them, and what success could look like. This in turn influenced how the rota (roster) was written, and what happened in team meetings and supervisions.

In this example, Carolynn and her team aligned purpose and performance and then aligned with people when looking at who supported Anne-Marie to deliver her perfect week.

Clarifying performance

Now that your team has developed its purpose statement and has reflected on what matters most to its members, you can clarify performance expectations and how you'll measure them in the context of your purpose.

As you answer the performance questions in this chapter you'll be creating and defining methods, measures and metrics. As stated earlier, this can be counter-cultural to many teams, but it's critical to success and enabling teams to recognise their good work and achievement.

We will look at each of these questions in turn:

- What does success look like?

- How can we know how well we are doing?

In this section you'll see examples of how teams have approached these questions with their members. A few – like one-page strategies and Starbursting – cover both questions, so we'll start with those.

ONE-PAGE STRATEGY

A one-page strategy aligns success from different perspectives with the processes to achieve that success, and how a team measures performance (your team's purpose, performance and process summary defined on one page). To develop this, you need to define what success looks like from different perspectives.

To demonstrate this alignment we re-introduce the example we shared in Chapter 2 of how a training team, Housing Associates, thought about its purpose.

Table 4.2 Housing Associates thinking about purpose

Our purpose in relation to people who attend our courses	Our purpose in relation to people who commission our courses	Our purpose in relation to our team	Our purpose in relation to the organisation
To help people develop the skills and knowledge they need to do their job.	To understand the outcomes they want to achieve from the training.	To support each other to deliver the best services possible to course participants and customers.	To deliver our services within budget in a way that reflects the organisation's mission, vision and values.
To deliver training in an engaging and creative way that respects the existing knowledge of staff.	To design a programme with clear aims and objectives to deliver outcomes.	To learn together, and continually improve the services we offer.	

Then they added what success would look like if they achieved their purpose (see Table 4.3).

Table 4.3 *Housing Associates – what does success look like?*

Success from different perspectives

Participants	Customers	Team	Organisation
Participants have new skills they can use in their workplace. Participants have new knowledge that's useful in their workplace. The training is engaging and builds on participants' knowledge.	The training achieves outcomes in an efficient and engaging way.	Feels supported. They learn together and continually improve their service.	Training is delivered to customer satisfaction within budget and in a way that reflects the company's values.

There are many ways that the impact of a training team can be measured, such as in-depth before and after evaluations of knowledge and skills; participant behaviour being observed in the workplace to see how it reflects the knowledge and skills taught on the course; or arranging interviews and focus groups.

However, the Housing Associates' team needed to find a way to measure their success that was proportionate and affordable and reflected what they were in control of and their sphere of influence. Other people – in this situation, it was managers – share the responsibility of how well staff put what they have learned into practice. Here are the measures they decided on, that are both doable and within their control.

Table 4.4 *Housing Associates – how will we know if we are successful?*

How will we know if we are successful?

Participants	Customers	Team	Organisation
The percentage of participants who score 70 per cent or more in our course follow-up evaluation (survey monkey) that state they have new skills and knowledge they can use in their workplace.	In our post-course evaluation the percentage of customers who rate us as good or excellent in response to the statement: 'The training achieved our outcomes.'	We review the support section in our one-page profile with our manager every quarter, and develop actions based on what is or is not working.	Delivering our service within budget.

cont.

Participants	Customers	Team	Organisation
The percentage of participants who score 70 per cent or more in relation to the training being engaging.		We have an annual whole-team person-centred review and agree on actions from this.	

As you can see, this is a combination of metrics (numbers) and other ways of measuring progress. It could be tempting to make the team section metrics based on counting the number of actions achieved. This, however, comes with a warning: measuring success this way creates a perverse incentive to set actions that are easily achieved. Instead, this team went for ensuring that a review takes place for each team member, that this is based on their one-page profile and, in particular, the support section, and that actions are agreed from this (in the belief that we can always improve how we support each other). To complete their one-page strategy, the team then added the processes that they would use to achieve success – the subject of the next chapter.

In 2010 two organisations – Southside Partnership (including Fanon) which supports people with learning disabilities, and people with mental health issues and Support for Living which predominantly supports people with learning disabilities – merged to form Certitude (previously mentioned in Chapter 1). The merger brought together two distinct cultures, but similar values, and the newly established leadership team wanted to communicate clearly what they were now working towards and how they wanted to measure their performance.

The leadership team includes Aisling, the CEO, Mark, the Human Resources Director, Sanjay, the Finance Director, Marianne, Director of Development, as well as three operational directors, Mary, Nicholas and Janette.

One of the first tasks of the new team was to create their individual one-page profiles and draw up a team one-page profile. Their next step was to bring together their newly revised mission statement and pull this into a one-page strategy as a way to summarise what success means in relation to the people they support, the staff and the business/organisation. The leadership team worked together to develop success statements, how they could use person-centred practices to achieve this success (process) and how they would measure this. They used information from a recent consultation with people they support, and developed and then refined a draft. They had this as an agenda item for two consecutive leadership team meetings in order to get to a draft that they were happy with, with Mark and Janette spending a few hours on it in between meetings. Once the leadership team was happy with that draft, they then consulted with a wide group of staff and managers. They had a 'strategy day' where they shared the work that the leadership team had been doing (one-page profiles and their leadership team one-page profile) with their strategy on a page, and also used the day to talk about the branding for the new organisation. Staff and managers gave helpful feedback on how the language could be simplified and Figure 4.1 is the third version, based on that feedback:

For Certitude, success meant it was invested in its workforce by:

- increasing scores in the management competency self-assessment Progress for Providers for Managers[32]
- increasing the percentage of staff who have received person-centred thinking training
- improving absenteeism.

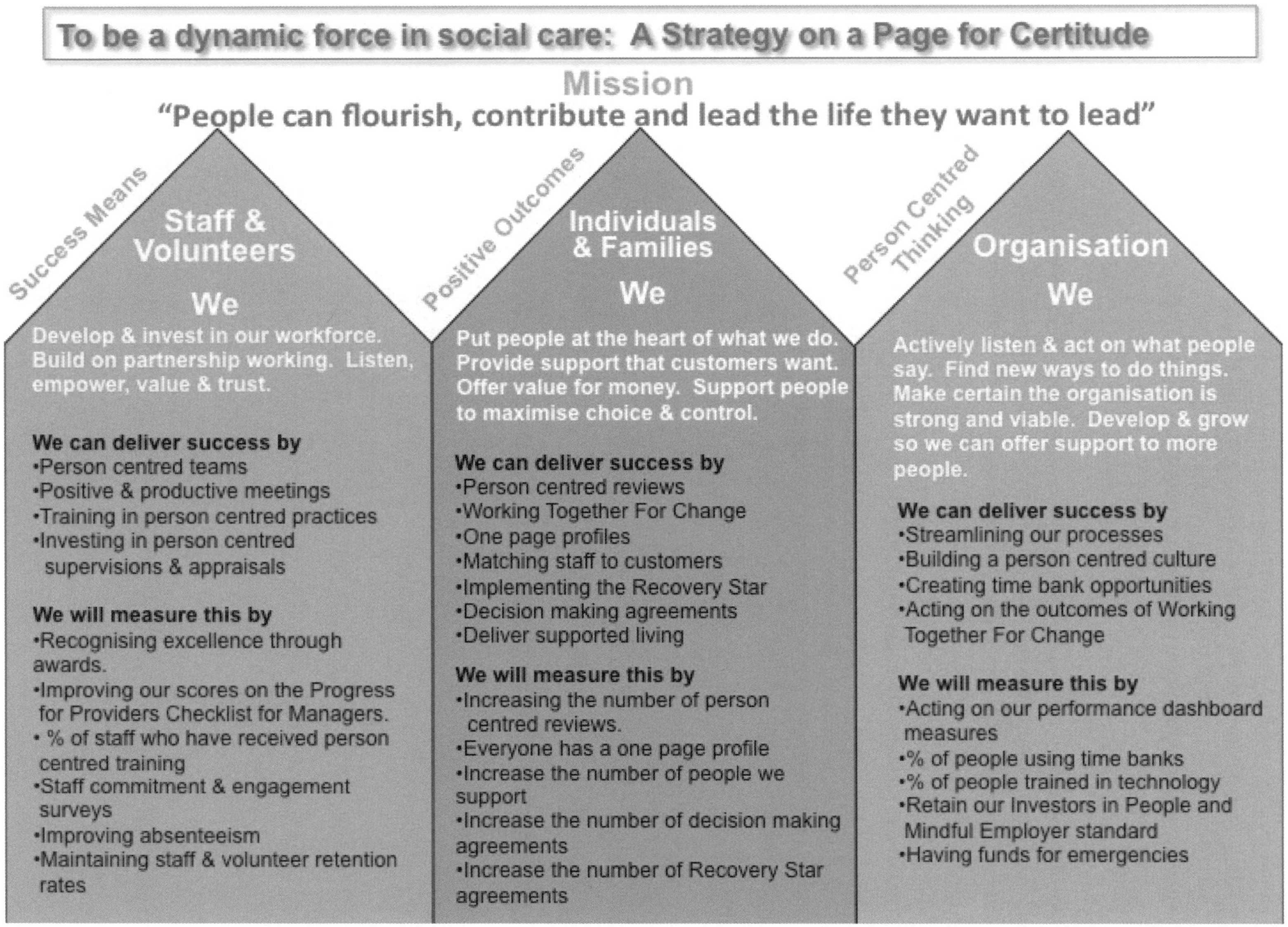

To be a dynamic force in social care: A Strategy on a Page for Certitude

Mission

"People can flourish, contribute and lead the life they want to lead"

Success Means — **Positive Outcomes** — **Person Centred Thinking**

Staff & Volunteers

We

Develop & invest in our workforce. Build on partnership working. Listen, empower, value & trust.

We can deliver success by
- Person centred teams
- Positive & productive meetings
- Training in person centred practices
- Investing in person centred supervisions & appraisals

We will measure this by
- Recognising excellence through awards.
- Improving our scores on the Progress for Providers Checklist for Managers.
- % of staff who have received person centred training
- Staff commitment & engagement surveys
- Improving absenteeism
- Maintaining staff & volunteer retention rates

Individuals & Families

We

Put people at the heart of what we do. Provide support that customers want. Offer value for money. Support people to maximise choice & control.

We can deliver success by
- Person centred reviews
- Working Together For Change
- One page profiles
- Matching staff to customers
- Implementing the Recovery Star
- Decision making agreements
- Deliver supported living

We will measure this by
- Increasing the number of person centred reviews.
- Everyone has a one page profile
- Increase the number of people we support
- Increase the number of decision making agreements
- Increase the number of Recovery Star agreements

Organisation

We

Actively listen & act on what people say. Find new ways to do things. Make certain the organisation is strong and viable. Develop & grow so we can offer support to more people.

We can deliver success by
- Streamlining our processes
- Building a person centred culture
- Creating time bank opportunities
- Acting on the outcomes of Working Together For Change

We will measure this by
- Acting on our performance dashboard measures
- % of people using time banks
- % of people trained in technology
- Retain our Investors in People and Mindful Employer standard
- Having funds for emergencies

Figure 4.1 Certitude's one-page strategy

The leadership team recognised that 'improving' or 'increasing' could be as little as 1 per cent, so they decided to get baseline data of where they currently were and set very specific targets for the percentage of improvements they wanted to see.

At their next meeting they focused on the measures to get a baseline on how they were performing so they could properly invest their HR team's resources in training and coaching well.

A one-page strategy is a way that a team at any level, or a project team, can summarise what success looks like from different perspectives, and how the team will measure this success, therefore addressing both of the performance questions.

STARBURSTING

Another unique approach that addresses both performance questions is Starbursting, a technique similar to brainstorming that enables a team to think about performance, consider available options, assess each question and rule out non-essential ideas.

A group of Workforce Investment Act (WIA) Youth Program Providers in California were attempting to clarify what programmes and services would be effective in providing youth with opportunities to compete successfully in the labour market and prepare them for higher education.

To assist them with this process, they were asked to think through questions that focused on who, what, where, when, why and how. This Starbursting process provided an opportunity for visualisation and helped to capture a picture of performance onto one page (see Figure 4.2).

Starbursting questions:

- Who will be involved and affected?

- What will success look like?

- Where will we be doing the project?

- When will the project be completed?

- Why are we doing this project?

- How will we know the project is complete and done well?

Starbursting brings together purpose and people as well as addressing what success looks like, and the responsibilities team members have to achieve it.[33]

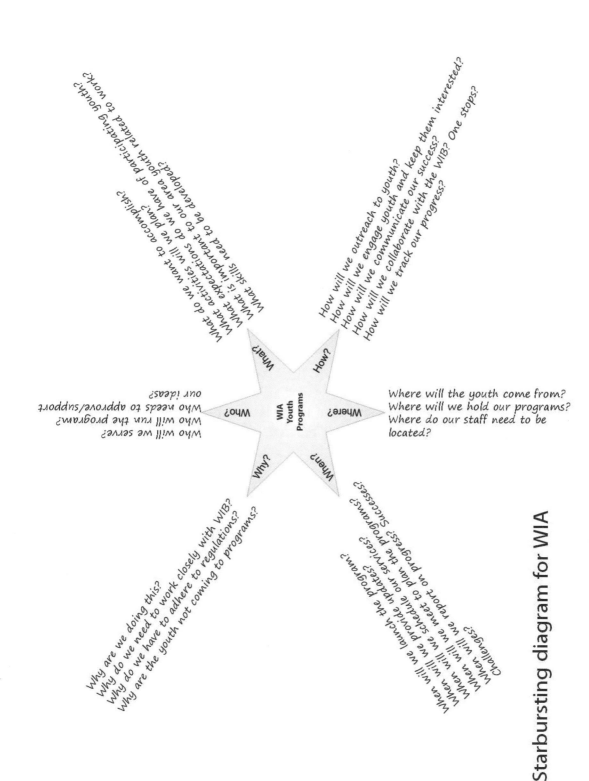

How will we outreach to youth?
How will we engage youth and keep them interested?
How will we communicate our success?
How will we collaborate with the WIB? One stops?
How will we track our progress?

What do we want to accomplish?
What activities will we plan?
What is important to our area youth?
What skills need to be developed?
What skills need to be developed for participating youth to work?

WIA Youth Programs

What?

How?

Where?

When?

Why?

Who?

Where will the youth come from?
Where will we hold our programs?
Where do our staff need to be located?

Who will we serve?
Who will run the program?
Who needs to approve/support our ideas?

When will we launch the program?
When will we provide the program?
When will we meet to schedule our services?
When will we meet to plan updates?
When will we report on progress? Successes? Challenges?

Why are we doing this?
Why do we need to work closely with WIB?
Why do we have to adhere to regulations?
Why are the youth not coming to programs?

Starbursting diagram for WIA

Figure 4.2 Starbursting diagram for WIA

Performance question 1: what does success look like?

So far we have looked at two ways to define success and think about how to measure this at a whole-team level. We also need to consider this at an individual level so that team members know what is expected of them – what their core responsibilities are and what competencies they need to have. In relation to core responsibilities, the main way to do this is by using a Doughnut. People work best when they know what is expected of them – so they have clear guidelines and the freedom to work within them, and know where they can experiment. This is where the Doughnut is helpful. A person-centred team has a culture of trust, empowerment and accountability.

THE DOUGHNUT

The Doughnut clarifies areas in your job where experimentation is not allowed and making mistakes can be an issue, and where experimentation and making mistakes are actively encouraged and celebrated.

Adapted from the work of Irish philosopher and organisational development author, Charles Handy, the Doughnut defines what a team will/will not do as it seeks to achieve its purpose and adhere to the organisation's core mission. This tool helps to answer the performance questions by arranging the tasks and work activity into those things that are core responsibilities, and which, if they were not performed or not performed well, would have serious consequences for the team or individual member. Also to be considered are those items around which the team can use some creativity and judgement in determining how the work is performed. These are areas where people are encouraged to try new things, take risks and make mistakes – this is where innovation happens. Finally, it is important to consider those activities or services that do not belong to the team and are beyond its scope of responsibility. Considering all three of these areas helps people to remain focused on the core mission and purpose of the team and avoid mission creep, which can be costly and ineffective (see Figure 4.3).

The Housing Associates training team looked at their success statements and thought together about what was a core responsibility that they could not mess with, and all the areas that they could experiment with and explore.

One of their success criteria was that the training was engaging, and built on participants' existing knowledge.

They decided that a core responsibility was to use a range of methods within their training that was best fitted to the material to deliver the specified outcomes. The other core responsibility was for trainers to share what they learned worked well with the rest of the team. In the creativity and judgement section, they decided that trainers could experiment with which methods they wanted to use, how they recorded what they learned about the effectiveness of different approaches, and when and how they shared it with the team. This gave the trainers lots of opportunity to experiment with different ways to meet the training objectives. What was core, that they could not experiment with, was changing the objectives. Within permission to experiment, there is permission to make mistakes and accept that not all new approaches will work brilliantly, but the core responsibility was to make sure that this learning was shared with the team, so they could build on each other's innovation and not repeat mistakes unnecessarily.

SHARED DOUGHNUTS

Once the performance expectations of the team have been established (what success looks like), a shared Doughnut can be created that reflects the core responsibilities of all team members, along with the areas where they're encouraged to use creativity and judgement to achieve performance goals and objectives. This can cover all aspects of performance, or can be shared with people from other teams who need to work together to achieve change.

Julie – a seven-year-old – attended a mainstream school and had special educational needs. The shared Doughnut example (see Figure 4.4) is around the support she needed from teachers and their assistants, the SENCO (special educational needs co-ordinator) and her parents.

A further example is from Enable Southwest, which is a provider organisation in the south west of Western Australia. It uses person-centred reviews to establish individual outcomes for people it supports. From this it uses the Doughnut to clarify the individual expectations of staff, and how responsibility is shared with the family to meet the outcome. Enable has been established for over 21 years and has been moving towards becoming authentically person-centred in its values, practice and, most importantly, the support offered to people who use its services. Part of this change has included using person-centred reviews.

The questions that the facilitator may ask in this part of the review are:

- What needs to happen to make sure that what is working in your life keeps happening?

- What needs to happen to change what is not working for you? What will your life look like if we have changed this (your outcomes)?

- What can we do together to enable you to move towards what is important in the future?

- How can we address each of the 'questions to answer'? What else do we need to learn?

We get to outcomes by both looking together at changing what is not working and thinking about what difference that would make; and how to move towards the life the person wants, and think about what is possible in a year. This is what this looked like for John (see Table 4.5).

★

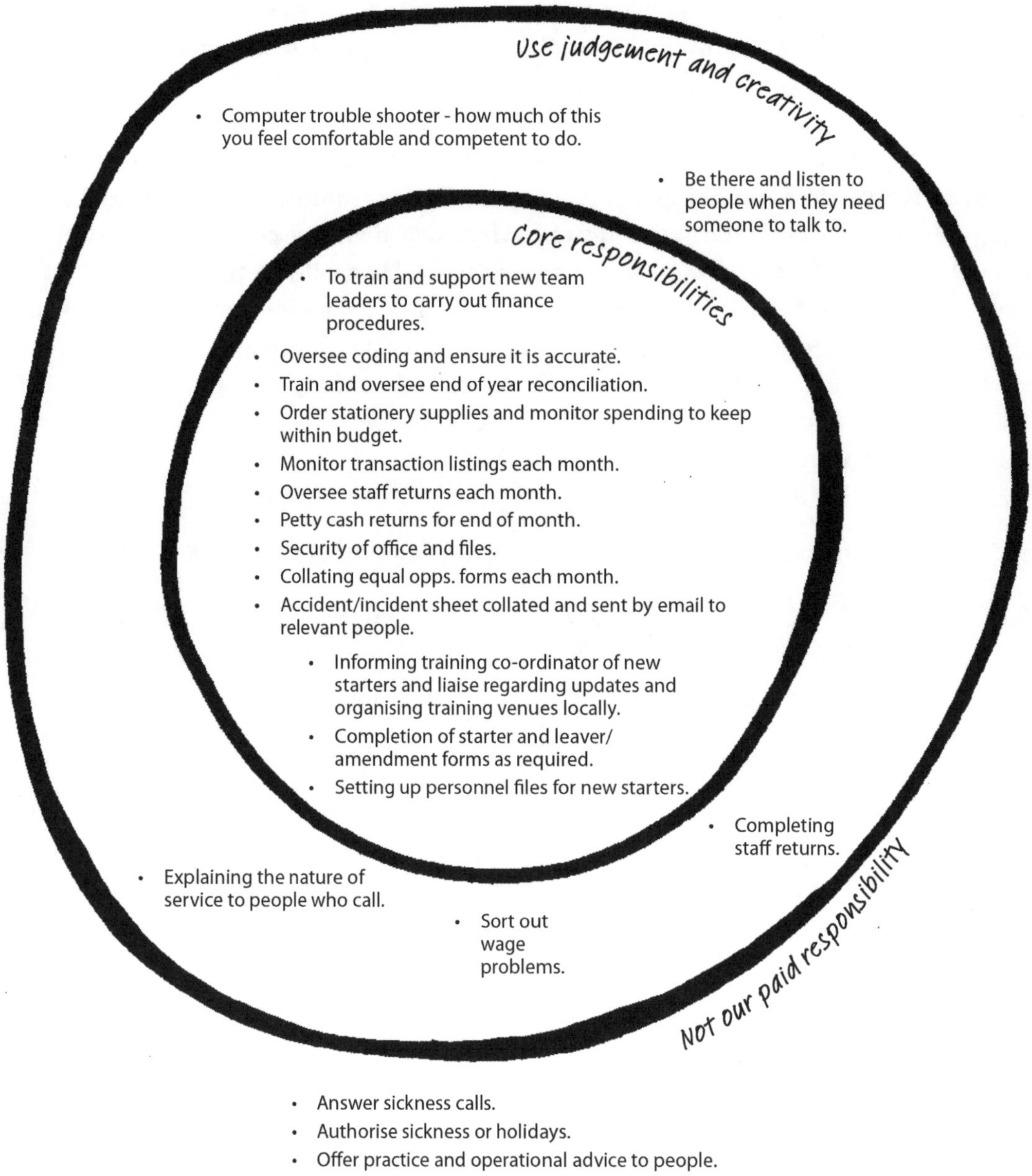
Use judgement and creativity
Computer trouble shooter - how much of this you feel comfortable and competent to do.
Be there and listen to people when they need someone to talk to.
Core responsibilities
To train and support new team leaders to carry out finance procedures.
Oversee coding and ensure it is accurate.
Train and oversee end of year reconciliation.
Order stationery supplies and monitor spending to keep within budget.
Monitor transaction listings each month.
Oversee staff returns each month.
Petty cash returns for end of month.
Security of office and files.
Collating equal opps. forms each month.
Accident/incident sheet collated and sent by email to relevant people.
Informing training co-ordinator of new starters and liaise regarding updates and organising training venues locally.
Completion of starter and leaver/ amendment forms as required.
Setting up personnel files for new starters.
Completing staff returns.
Explaining the nature of service to people who call.
Sort out wage problems.
Not our paid responsibility
Answer sickness calls.
Authorise sickness or holidays.
Offer practice and operational advice to people.

Figure 4.3 The Doughnut

	Core Responsibilities	Where you can use creativity and judgement	Not your responsibility
Class Teacher	Share information to keep this plan updated and meet with Mum every 6 weeks to add/change information (including information from the learning logs). Setting and helping Julie to achieve her targets.	Ways to record new information – e.g. writing directly on the plan, in a notebook etc. Adapting the learning log with the teaching assistants and Julie's Mum.	Arranging for Julie to play with her friends outside of school.
Learning Support Assistants	Share information with the class teacher to keep this plan updated. Use learning logs every day to share with Mum what we are learning. Not to use phonics – this does not work for Julie. Using the visual timetable. Ensuring that Julie stays warm (particularly in very cold weather). Ensuring that Julie takes her medication (there is a medication chart for Julie in the medical room).	Exploring other ways to help Julie understand what is going to happen next, in addition to her visual timetable.	Arranging for Julie to play with her friends outside of school.
SENCO	Arranging Julie's review meetings. Recording and sharing the actions from these meetings.	Exploring different ways to have these meetings so that they include Julie and everyone can share their views, for example, using 'working and not working from different perspectives'. Explore whether this 9 – 3.15 plan can replace the IEP.	
Head Teacher	Reviewing Julie's statement.	How this is recorded.	
Family	Share information to keep this plan updated.	Supporting Julie in her friendships and relationships outside of school.	

Figure 4.4 Example of school shared Doughnut

Table 4.5 John – what is working/not working?

Perspective	Working	Not working
John	See my friend Jim every month or so.	
Mum	I feel John is safe. Seeing him a couple of times a month.	Sometimes there is inconsistency in the staff team.
Staff team supporting John	John seems to love football and watching matches on the TV, and going to matches with staff when he can.	John only sees his mum, Jim and the team. He does not have other people in his life.

What is important to John in the future?: To have his own place, and be connected to people.

Outcome: John to have more people in his life (other than staff and family).

How do we go from this, to staff knowing what they need to do on a day-to-day basis – our performance expectations for them? We also need to consider how we assist others potentially to take on tasks that are beyond the scope of a service provider.

To make sure that everyone is clear about their roles and responsibilities in achieving outcomes, we use a Doughnut, but 'split' it, so it becomes a shared Doughnut, so that we can look at different roles in achieving the outcomes. The following sections can be done as a separate implementation meeting.

Outcome

John to have more people in his life (other than staff and family)

Table 4.6 Shared responsibilities for supporting John

Person	My core responsibilities	Where I can use judgement and be creative	What is not my (paid) responsibility
Support worker	To always be on the lookout for potential connections. To introduce John to other people in a positive, confident and friendly way. Support John to keep and enhance his existing relationship with Jim.	To decide with John when to invite someone to have coffee/go for a drink. Thinking with John about whether he wants to spend more time with Jim and how he wants to stay in touch.	Whether the person becomes John's friend.

Co-ordinator	Develop the roster to make sure that John is supported by the same person, at the same time to go to the three new places on his community map.	How to support the team to reflect on their learning – for example, learning logs, four-plus-one.
	Match staff interests and hobbies to these places as much as possible.	
	Support the team to learn from what they are trying and learning with John.	
John	To decide who I am interested in getting to know more.	
Mum	To check with John that he is happy with how things are going.	

Performance question 2: how can we know how well we are doing?

AGREEING ON INDIVIDUAL PERFORMANCE TARGETS

A one-page strategy clearly identifies what success looks like from different perspectives within the context of a team's purpose. The Doughnut drills down to address what the core responsibilities are and where a team can be creative in order to achieve success.

The next focus is deciding what this means for individuals since different teams use different language. They may be called targets, goals or objectives, but however they are described they clearly agree on what the person is going to be doing and the level or performance or improvement that's expected.

Targets are typically set together by a team leader and a supervisor working together to achieve the same goals. Usually targets are set by you and the person in supervision. The research here is surprising – that when people set their own targets, they set tougher targets and they are more likely to achieve them.[34]

A team of instructors had decided together that success meant that training was engaging, and built on participants' existing knowledge. From this, the team developed a Doughnut to clarify what they must to do make it engaging. This included using a variety of methods in the training, for example, scenarios, exercises and experiential learning to deliver the outcomes.

Tony, one of the instructors, wanted to set himself the target of moving from the three methods that he usually used to exploring two other approaches (for example, *Prezi* instead of *PowerPoint*, and instead of sharing scenarios with slides, using video instead). He also wanted to go beyond the team target of a 70 per cent score on his training being engaging; he wanted to set a performance target for himself of 75 per cent.

These would be reviewed together in person-centred supervision, which we describe in the Process chapter.

The Expectation Arrow

Another way to clarify expectations in delivering performance is to use the Expectation Arrow, which is based on the concept that team performance is built from the results of team actions. It's human nature to want to be successful; therefore, an employee won't approach a task thinking they're going to do a poor job. Which begs the question, why do people sometimes do poorly in their work? In part it's because they didn't have a clear understanding of what was really being asked of them, and may have had a different concept of what a 'good job' means.

The Expectation Arrow addresses three key elements to help people understand the desired outcome of their efforts, the motivating factors of their work and the level of quality that will define their success.

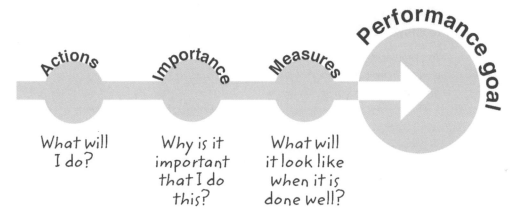

Figure 4.5 The Expectation Arrow

ACTIONS: WHAT WILL I DO?

Ask yourself 'What is the action and service I'll complete, or the product I'll deliver?' If you're a team member, make sure you understand exactly what you're being asked to do. If you're a supervisor or team leader, make sure you clearly understand the instructions.

Don, the development director of a high school music and arts support organisation, was in the midst of a fundraising campaign for the music teacher's salary, new uniforms, and band and choir competition travel. As he organised teams to conduct donor outreach, he provided clear expectations to Carla, one of the volunteer team members:

> I'd like you to call the 300 donors on this list within the next two months to update their donor profile and request a contribution to our fundraising campaign.

IMPORTANCE: WHY IS IT IMPORTANT THAT I DO THIS?

When you align a work request with something meaningful, and to something important to those affected by the work activity, you increase the likelihood the team member will achieve the desired performance.

Framing work expectations gives meaning to people's efforts, tells them why the result is important, and links what they do with your organisation's goals.

Don further clarified his request:

> Carla, the school funding for the music programme has been cut by 50 per cent, making it more important than ever that we reach out to our community. If we are not able to raise 50 per cent of the music programme budget for the upcoming academic year, we risk losing the music teacher and the entire music programme.
>
> Our donors really value music education and they appreciate how much the students contribute to the cultural vitality of our community. A personal phone call will allow us to connect with them in a meaningful way and give each donor an opportunity to make a significant difference to our students, our school and our community. I know how dedicated you have been to supporting the ongoing operations of the band and choir programmes, and your ability to engage people seems like a good fit for this job.

MEASURES: WHAT WILL IT LOOK LIKE WHEN IT IS DONE WELL?

Criteria such as quantity, quality, cost, time and degree of impact can be applied to help visualise the finished programme or service, and how it will be evaluated (the outcome). It's also helpful to know how close the person must get to the desired result to be considered successful.

> Carla, there are 300 people on this list. Success involves making a minimum of 75 phone calls per week, using this script when you conduct your calls, completing all of the fields in the donor profile spreadsheet and asking each donor for a contribution amount based on their previous donation level as indicated in their profile. Our overall team performance goal is to raise $75,000 by June 30.

When communicating expectations, the 'command and control' approach needs to be avoided as it inhibits engagement. Person-centred teams rely on listening, understanding, open dialogue, honouring what's important and building on member strengths that lead to desired results.

This example demonstrates how Don effectively engaged team members as he communicated performance expectations during the fundraising campaign.

- *State the expectation clearly and completely* by informing the team members what the results, measures and context are for the tasks.

  > Our organisation depends on strong relationships with our financial contributors, which means that donor profiles must be completed satisfactorily during the first call. This makes donors feel valued. Our new minimum standard for all campaign calling reps is now going to be that 98 per cent of calls will result in a donor profile completed accurately on the first call. 'Complete' means no additional follow-up is required with the donor for profile information.

- *Seek ideas from the team.* Ask questions…listen…understand.

  > We've had problems meeting our fundraising goals in the past. What do you think could be the cause? And what do you think we can do to make sure we meet our new goal to close the budget deficit?
  >
  > That's interesting. So, based on your experience, you think we should…?

- *Confirm understanding.* You and the team members should have the same picture of what the result looks like when it's well done.

Let's make sure we're saying the same thing. How many donors are you aiming to connect within weeks one and two?' *Agree on expected results.* Make sure the team thinks the performance expectation is appropriate and realistic.

Does meeting our new minimum standard in two-week increments make sense to you?

When you say you'll 'give it a try' I get the feeling you're not sure. Am I right?

What do you feel is realistic and appropriate?

Let's meet in one month to check on progress. In the meantime, call me if you have any questions or run into any obstacles.

Once the desired performance has been identified, it can be used as part of individual performance meetings and recorded on a performance development support plan.

Table 4.7 *Performance development support plan*

Performance development support plan

Date: Date to review:

Team member:

Performance goal (Action): What will I do and by when?

Importance: Why is it important to do this?

Measure of success: What will it look like when it is done well?

Support: How do I want to be supported in order to be successful?

Employee objectives (milestones) to make progress towards this goal

1. What	By when	How well	Support
2. What	By when	How well	Support

Manager actions/agreements to support progress towards this goal

1. What	By when	How well	Support
2. What	By when	How well	Support

Manager: _____   Employee: _____

Getting started

Defining performance converts the abstract concepts described in the team purpose statement into concrete, observable events or activities that can be measured or evidenced.

Performance helps to align the team's purpose with its daily work activities. Performance indicators build accountability and keep the team focused on continuous improvement for the benefit of the people served by the team. The team and individuals can then decide which processes will be needed to achieve expected results. Here are some considerations when you are getting started in thinking about this with your team.

ANSWER THE WHY? QUESTION BEFORE YOU START

Accountability and specifying what 'good' looks like can be counter-cultural in many organisations. If you sense that could be the case for your organisation or company, you'll need to explore the problems and address team concerns or objections before starting on a project.

WHAT WORKS FOR YOUR TEAM? LOOKING FORWARD OR BACKWARDS?

You can move from purpose to performance by imagining what has already happened; or you look backwards by imagining the customers and/or people you support having the lives they want. For example, you can say to your team:

> Imagine you've awakened from a long sleep and it's now three years into the future. The team is doing an amazing job and delivering everything in the purpose statement. Ask yourselves the following questions:
>
> - What is happening?
>
> - What can you see in the lives of the customers or people we support?
>
> - What do you see the team doing?
>
> - What are management and trustees pleased with?
>
> - What will be different as a result of us performing well?
>
> - What else would we notice? What would others notice?
>
> Now we're going to take all that information and brainstorm clear, specific success statements.

HAVE A CLEAR LINE OF SIGHT FROM PURPOSE TO WHAT SUCCESS LOOKS LIKE

The more specific you are about what success looks like, the easier it will be to decide how to measure it. Make sure there is a clear line of sight between success and what you plan to measure, then test it with other people (the notion that if it seems logical that success means this, it makes sense to measure that).

Positive Futures, a provider organisation in Northern Ireland committed to delivering person-centred and personalised support, sees success for staff as the hiring and retention of 'great staff and volunteers'. To measure how you 'keep' staff and volunteers, the metric naturally chosen is staff and volunteer retention rates.

CHOOSE DOABLE AND PROPORTIONATE MEASURES

The best measures are data that you already collect, but that is rarely the case for all your success statements. Where it is possible to use existing data, as Positive Futures has done in the above example, then this is very helpful. There is always a danger of putting more effort into measures than the time and energy that people have for delivering the results in the first place. So choose ways of knowing how well you are doing that are a reasonable reflection of the time and energy that it is possible to invest. It is better to start with one or two good ones, and then increase if you need more information on how well you are doing, than start with a raft of measures that feels overwhelming.

BALANCE METRICS WITH 'SOFT DATA'

Don't think the only indicator about how well the team is doing is numerical data. It can be combined with learning about what is/isn't working from different perspectives, compliments and complaint information, and stories of success and change.

When Stockport Council, Borough Care Ltd and HSA started to explore what personalisation could look like for 43 people living with dementia at Bruce Lodge, they agreed on a set of metrics to measure success. They quickly saw that they needed a better balance with soft data, so they arranged for a story to be filmed each month to capture people's changes, and used comment cards for families, staff and professionals to help inform the team about how they were doing.

AGREE ON CORE RESPONSIBILITIES OR PERFORMANCE STANDARDS

As you start looking at what team core responsibilities are, make sure that every member is involved in the decision making on what those responsibilities might be. If they're handed down from management rather than co-created with your team, you'll get little buy-in, and compliance instead of clarity of accountability.

Recording the information in the person-centred team plan

So far, the person-centred team plan should have a purpose statement or graphic and one-page staff profiles. You might also have a synthesis of what's important and how to best support the team. Now you can add information about performance to the emerging plan, such as:

One-page strategy. This can have the purpose at the top, then success from different perspectives and how you'll know how well you're doing. In the next chapter you will add the processes that you will use to deliver success. Certitude's leadership team started with their individual one-page profiles and then developed a one-page team plan. To this they added their one-page strategy.

Summarise what success looks like and how you will deliver this. If you used the Expectation Arrow or Starbursting as a way to think about success with your team, pull out the key messages from this and put this in your person-centred team plan.

Add a second page to each individual's one-page profile. We call this a one-page profile plus. We keep the one-page profile with its usual headings, like an executive summary, and then each team member has further 'plus' pages. You could create a second page with information about each individual performance expectations and how these will be measured. This is useful if people have different roles within your team, for example, a community health team of different professionals.

Add a team Doughnut to communicate core responsibilities. In the HSA person-centred team plan we have core responsibilities for each aspect of our work together, and where people can use their creativity and their own initiative.

In Figure 4.6 you can see how the Oxnard Children's Team added the core responsibilities to their team plan. They added these statements after doing a team Doughnut exercise.

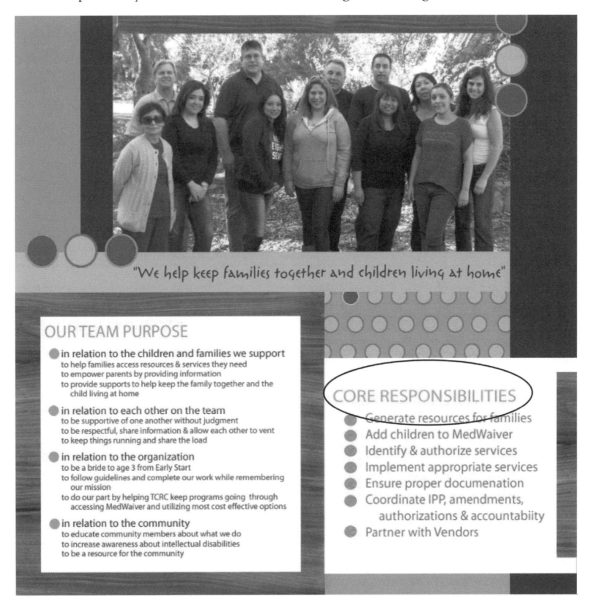

Figure 4.6 Core responsibilities for the Oxnard Children's Team

For some people this is where we move from 'warm' (and some cynically say 'fluffy') statements about why we are here and who is in the team and how we can support each other, to hard-edged metrics for measuring success.

It is crucial that all team members have a 'clear line of sight' from the purpose, through to what success looks like and how we know how well we are doing in performance. In the next chapter we return to the gifts and strengths of people to look at how we align the processes within the team with the people within the team, to be sure to deliver great performance.

Table 4.8 *Performance checklist*

Performance checklist	Strongly disagree	Disagree	Agree	Strongly agree
I know what is expected of us as a team.	☐	☐	☐	☐
I know what is expected of me.	☐	☐	☐	☐
I know what team success looks like and how this will be evaluated.	☐	☐	☐	☐
I know what our core responsibilities are in relation to our team purpose and overall mission of the organisation.	☐	☐	☐	☐
We have a record in our person-centred team plan of what success means.	☐	☐	☐	☐
We have a record in our team plan of how we can know how successful we are.	☐	☐	☐	☐
Our ways of measuring success are proportionate and we can do them within our resources.	☐	☐	☐	☐

Chapter 5

Process

How one undertakes a project, how one plans for it, and how the people affected are engaged by it are as important as the outcome.

Susan Jurow

Process is a series of actions or changes that take place in a defined manner to bring about a result. As Susan Jurow – author of *Change: The Importance of Process* – suggests, the impact of how people go about their work is just as important as the change they're trying to create.[35]

When teams use intentional person-centred practices, they become equipped to build positive relationships and maintain a culture that keeps people at the heart of the team's actions, and encourages trust, empowerment and accountability.

We've answered the 'Why are we here?', 'Who are you?' and 'What does success look like?' questions. Process is the 'how' question, so we'll now focus on delivery and how it can be achieved.

Process questions

In this chapter you will answer two questions about how your team works together and the processes that you use to deliver:

- How will we work together?

- How will we deliver success?

We want you to find ways to enable and support your team to work together in ways that reflect a person-centred culture and what is important to your team. However, this alone is not sufficient – the way you work together must effectively deliver what you have agreed as your performance expectations.

Here are the person-centred practices that can help you address the questions around your team's processes.

Table 5.1 Addressing the process questions

Process question	You will have finished this section when...	Helpful tools
How will we work together?	You understand formal and informal rules. You can apply Positive and Productive Meetings practices of rounds and agenda development.	Ground rules and guidelines. Rounds.

cont.

Process question	You will have finished this section when...	Helpful tools
	You know how decisions are made.	Agenda development.
		Decision-making agreements.
	You know how you'll be involved in decisions that affect you.	
How will we deliver success?	You know how to get the best fit between roles and tasks and the people on your team.	Matching.
		Steps to success.
	You know how to move from success to delivering it.	Person-centred supervision.
	You know how to use person-centred supervision to support performance.	

What does 'process' mean?

Process defines how a team works together, how the work gets done and how decisions are made. It includes clarity about who will do what, when and how and it defines systems and practices that keep the team focused on the five Ps of a person-centred team.

This section will help you think about:

- What do we want to agree on how we work together?

- How can we be clear about how we make decisions together?

- How can we have meetings that are effective, productive and positive?

- How can we get the best fit between an individual's talents and interests and the tasks the team has to do?

- How can we plan for success?

- How can I support my team members to deliver success?

The processes chosen by a team are influenced by the team purpose, values and personality styles, and the strengths and gifts of members. Person-centred teams put values into practice by designing processes that support clear responsibility, shared decision making and working to team members' strengths. We think that how a team gets together – what happens in meetings – is a microcosm of the culture of the team. We shall explore this further when we look at the process of team meetings and how to make them both positive and productive. Before we look at this, let's think more about the culture that you may want to see in all of your team processes and why this is important.

Why is process important?

Each day we perform individual tasks without thinking about processes. When we organise our desk, when we sort emails, when we start our work projects for the day, it is possible that we could use a different approach each time we engage in a particular task and not be concerned with matters of consistency. Some performance standards can be met without attention to process.

When we move from individual tasks to team tasks that need to be performed by different people at different times, or performed on behalf of many different people, it is important to consider process for several reasons. Clarity and consistency of process will maximise the team's ability to successfully deliver success. Attention to process contributes to overall team health, trust, empowerment and accountability.

OVERALL TEAM HEALTH

When implementing person-centred team-work the intent is to work smarter, not harder. In reality, it takes the same amount of time to complete a work objective regardless of whether person-centred practices have been implemented. If the team isn't engaged and committed, they may have questions and concerns that can make the project longer and more difficult than it needs to be. Therefore, process is critical to a project's long-term success and the team's overall health.

Each project or initiative leaves behind an impression: did it support and promote a healthy team culture or did it leave behind hurt feelings, mistrust and cynical discontent? Person-centred teams anticipate the relationship-building and education that must take place in order to engage everyone involved and for the process to succeed. It should leave people excited about the potential of positive change because they were an inherent part of creating it. New skills and greater trust develop, which increases the likelihood that the next initiative can take place more swiftly and efficiently.

A question for the team becomes: how do you want to invest your time? At the front end to engage others through consensus-building to increase chances of a positive outcome? Or at the back end to repair relationships and clean up the fall-out of frustration and discontent?

In his work with person-centred organisations, Michael Smull describes the importance of respect, trust and partnership as 'markers of a person-centred culture'. We agree that trust is essential, and see respect and partnership as part of a culture rooted in empowerment and accountability.

Trust: Trust is a major component of positive interpersonal relationships, as a strong foundation in trust contributes to improved team performance. 'Build trust and you speed up everything,' says Stephen Covey in *The Speed of Trust.*[36]

Processes that define what is respectful, fair and equitable among team members support the development of trust. They construct how the team handles everyday and recurring actions like communications, decision making and conflict resolution.

> Arne and Lucy work for the same agency and both want to take time off during the same two-week period. However, it is important that one of them stays at the work site to provide coverage. Without a process in place to clarify how to request vacation time and how decisions are made, they may think that favouritism factors into the decision.

When employees supported by the organisation perceive unfair treatment or inequitable services, they can become sceptical and lose trust. Lack of fairness (whether real or perceived) in a decision can lead to significant tension between team members.

Empowerment: Team processes translate values into action. The way team members work together to deliver their purpose lets others know if they are walking the walk and/or talking the talk. When work processes encourage employees to contribute to planning, problem solving and decision making, it's more likely that employees will be satisfied and committed for the long-run.

> Employees at the Tri-Counties Regional Center are encouraged to participate in an agency-wide operations committee to share information, discuss issues and ideas and contribute to decision making. They're also supported with a performance review process that encourages staff to identify annual and other job-related goals.
> Employee development is supported through training, coaching and conversations about what is/ isn't working for the employees. These processes are enactments of a shared value of empowerment.

Accountability: Clear and compelling processes that deliver the purpose and reflect performance standards are imperative, and need to be aligned at organisational, team and individual levels. When a team focuses on its purpose it is doing good. But doing good does not guarantee that the team is doing good *well*. An organisation cannot survive on mission-driven passion alone. Clear processes that reflect person-centred values contribute to doing things well. That consistency of practice gives employees a sense of comfort in knowing what to expect and what they can rely on. Team members can 'trust the process', allowing them to focus on work activities that contribute to excellent individual and team outcomes.

PROCESSES TO DELIVER SUCCESS

Now that you're clear about purpose, the people in your team and what performance is expected, it's time to help your team think about how it will work together. This ranges from establishing team guidelines, to thinking about meetings and decision making.

Process question 1: how will we work together?

One-page profiles and one-page team profiles serve an important function in helping to determine processes that will work well for the team. Look at what is important to individuals and the team as a whole. Here are some ways to embed processes in your team-work to reflect the information shared in one-page profiles.

GUIDELINES

Different teams use different labels such as values and principles, detailed guidelines or ground rules. All are summaries of how a team works together.

You do not want this to become the team rulebook. Principles work better than rules because a rule has to be obeyed, and to do that, you are expected to suspend your judgement.[37] With a principle, we expect people to be thoughtful in how they apply it. Rules encourage people to work to the letter of the law and not within the spirit of the law. Think about this in relation to claiming expenses. Most organisations, and indeed the Houses of Parliament, have clear rules on what and how to claim for these. During 2009 there was a scandal around the ridiculous expenses that some MPs were claiming. Henry Stewart suggests this was not an abuse of trust, 'The main defence that MPs gave was that they had obeyed the rules. This was an example of how having rules got in the way of good judgement. The question became not "Is this a morally acceptable use of taxpayers' money?" but "Does it fit within the rules?"' (Stewart, p.37). The solution is transparency. Henry goes on to say, 'The best pressure to make an MP claim only appropriate expenses is not a more detailed set of rules but the knowledge that whatever they claim will be made public, and they will have to defend what they have done to the voters.'

Guidelines are agreements that describe how team members work together. Teams often start by agreeing to specific ground rules, usually during meetings, and build from there. When issues arise and are confronted, the learning can be added to the guidelines or ground rules. Some people think that this is unnecessary, and you simply need to apply what is called The Golden Rule and to treat everyone as you would like to be treated yourself. Not in a person-centred team. Here is an example, from Helen's blog:

> When I worked in services supporting people with learning disabilities in Manchester, I worked with a team using person-centred planning. The team did some excellent work in providing very person-centred support, with two people who did not use words to speak. As well as giving them direct feedback and praise, I wanted their efforts and success to be rewarded and acknowledged. I thought that the best way to do this was to get the Head of Service to write to them to express her appreciation.
>
> The next time I spent time with the team, I was surprised that they had not seemed very interested in the letter. I was disappointed. We started to have a conversation about appreciation and I asked them 'What does appreciation look like to you?' They told me that what they really would have liked would have been to share what they had tried and learned with their peers. We arranged for two of the team to talk at the next staff development forum to do this. I learned an important lesson about assuming that what would have felt like appreciation to me (being recognised by the Head of Service), is what being appreciated feels like to other people.
>
> This made me realise that 'treat people as you would like to be treated' does not work when you are trying to be person-centred with staff. You need to find out how people want to be treated and not assume that it is the same as you.

To create ground rules or guidelines, one-page profiles can be reviewed for common themes (i.e., support, trust, follow-through, accountability, flexibility, etc.). Ask the team to identify the top three that are most important, then what it looks like when they are present at work. What would they need to make those points consistently present in the way the team works together?

> A team of service co-ordinators were experiencing internal tensions during staff meetings and decided to create some ground rules. They identified Respect, Trust and Positive Communication (RTPC) as the three items that mattered most to be effective, productive and well supported. After they wrote the three headings at the top of a flipchart, they set down what it could look like when the RTPC characteristics are present. Once the lists were generated, time was allotted for questions and answers.
>
> Each member was given five dots to place on points they believed to be most critical to the team's success, which allowed participants to immediately see where they were in sync.
>
> They took the top five items and agreed to seven guidelines that everyone would agree to follow. Whenever possible statements were framed in the positive (i.e., 'We will be on time' is far more effective than 'We will not be late'). This same process can be used to clarify agreements among team members related to how they get their work done.

Their team guidelines:

- We will check in to give everyone the opportunity to be heard.

- If we aren't able to resolve issues during a meeting, we commit to identifying the next step(s) using a constructive framework.

- Emotional/heated statements will be acknowledged and we will move on (or the group will collaboratively decide to continue the discussion).

- When we have questions, concerns or conflicts about individuals or work issues, we will include them in the conversation.

- We will check assumptions with the source.

- Only one person will speak at a time (we all have permission to remind people when they're out of order).

- We will check for understanding with one another.

Here is another example from an administration team who looked at each other's *good and bad days*, and came up with this list as a way for the whole team to have more good days:

- Ensure that the safe key is kept in the office.

- Make sure that we have tea/coffee and sugar, and that all the cups are washed the night before.

- Return files to where they belong at the end of the day.

- Let us know where you are, and if you plan to be out of the office use the wipe-off board to let us know.

- Pass on messages the same day.

Happy Computers has a four-page guidance document that sets down principles for its trainers. One core principle is simply 'Don't tell when you can ask'. As with all person-centred practices, good information on paper is only useful if it's applied and periodically revisited.

> The Santa Ynez Valley Humane Society Board of Directors in Santa Barbara, California, found a creative way to remain accountable to their team ground rules.
>
> As Mary Beth worked with the board, she learned that one area of struggle was around behaviour during meetings when members got derailed by talking over one another, interrupting and getting side-tracked by irrelevant content. To remedy this they developed meeting agreements on how they should work together, which helped for a while. But they still struggled to break old habits of getting off track and had a hard time holding each other accountable for the new agreements.
>
> Darcy, a board member and staff veterinarian, created laminated cards with photos of sheltered animals and attached them to the top of paint sticks. She had each board member pick one of the 'animal puppets' at the beginning of the meeting. If a board member had to be reminded about the meeting guidelines, anyone could wave the puppet as a friendly reminder.
>
> The basket of animal puppets is now an integral part of every meeting – a fun, harmless and creative solution that linked the self-improvement efforts of the board to the organisation's mission.

Develop Positive and Productive Meetings

As the example above shows, meetings are a vital process to get things right. It can be shocking to discover how many hours people spend in meetings each week and how little value they add.

> Senior leaders report spending 50 per cent or more of their time in meetings, and many claim that two-thirds of meetings end before participants can make important decisions. Not surprisingly, 85 per cent of executives surveyed in a Bain and Company study were dissatisfied with the efficiency and effectiveness of their organisation's meetings. (M Mankins and J Davis-Peccoud 2011)[38]

Every team has different struggles, but certain themes consistently emerge:

- People don't feel listened to.

- Agendas are too full.

- Certain individuals dominate discussions.

- Meeting are boring.

- At the end of meetings, people are unclear about what was agreed to and what they need to do because this wasn't recorded properly.

- The Chair does everything.

Many organisations have used *Positive and Productive Meetings* as a way to start to move towards a person-centred culture and delivering personalised services, and Michael Smull describes *Positive and Productive Meetings* as a key way to achieve person-centred cultural change.[39]

Positive and Productive Meetings[40] embed person-centred principles into meetings. They bring together elements of NLP (Neuro-linguistic Programming) (focus on outcomes) and creating a Thinking Environment (Nancy Kline, *Time to Think* 1998)[41] and components of person-centred teams (working to strengths and sharing roles). *Positive and Productive Meetings* are based on three simple guiding principles. Teams that want to work together positively and productively must:

- have a clear purpose for each meeting and an outcome for each agenda item

- have a process and an environment where people are listened to and think for themselves

- work to people's strengths and share responsibility for different roles in meetings.

This is a fresh approach to meetings that uses a person-centred approach and focuses on sharing roles and responsibilities in meetings and ensuring that roles reflect people's gifts and talents. *Positive and Productive Meetings* require clarity over decision making, and clear, outcome-focused, timed agendas that enable people to think together, make decisions and not just use meetings as a way to share information. The meeting process ensures that everyone is listened to and contributes to decision making.

ROUNDS

We were first introduced to rounds through the work of Nancy Kline and *Time to Think*. We recommend this book and Nancy's work to learn more about creating a thinking environment together. Rounds give everyone an uninterrupted chance to contribute their ideas and opinions on a focused question. They ensure that everyone's contributions are heard. A round creates an opportunity for people to both think for themselves and build on each other's ideas.

Every *Positive and Productive Meeting* opens and closes with a round. Rounds are also used within the agenda to generate ideas and get feedback from everyone throughout the meeting, particularly when the discussion is bogged down or being dominated by one or two personalities.

Opening rounds always start with the same question – 'What has gone well since we last met?' You can add 'at home and at work', but don't get more creative than this! The purpose of an opening round is to enable everyone to share something that is going well. Nancy explains that the mind thinks best in the presence of full information. As meetings will often focus on problems and what is not working, starting with something that is working well balances this.

An opening round is a great way to connect people on a personal level and helps them to separate from their previous activity and focus on being mindful and present for the meeting.

It also helps to shift brain chemistry.[42, 43] We feel what we think! When people think about something unpleasant they tend to become tense and angry. When people think about something positive, they become happier! It is that simple.

An important principle with rounds is equality. To achieve this you can either suggest that people take one or two minutes each, or remind people how much time there is for this round and ask them to be mindful of this when they have their turn.

An opening round gives everyone at the meeting an opportunity to speak. Everyone listens without interrupting and pays attention to the speaker. The facilitator gently reminds people about having an 'uninterrupted round' if people start to comment or talk.

Lightning rounds are an effective way to get contributions from large groups and to save time in a busy agenda. These follow the format of a typical round, but are faster! Meeting participants are limited to five or ten words to summarise their thoughts. Lightning rounds inspire quick thinking and creativity and should be used selectively as a way to get input. They do not create an opportunity for people to think things through or build on each other's ideas.

Examples of possible lightning round questions:

'What is one word that describes what you are thinking or feeling about where this discussion is heading?'

'Can you tell us in ten seconds or less, what you believe to be a next step forward?'

Generative rounds are a great way to hear from everyone, generate ideas and allow creative solutions to emerge as ideas build on the input of others.

> I (Mary Beth) was at a statewide eLearning Summit, where 25 training managers gathered from all over California to practise using new eLearning software to develop online learning content. When we arrived at the summit we learned that the venue did not have wireless internet capability and could not accommodate a hardwire connection for all participants.
>
> Suddenly we had 25 unhappy participants. Some were quick to criticise, while others were quick to make unilateral decisions. Everyone had something to voice, mostly frustration! As people tried to have their perspectives acknowledged and their suggestions considered, voices began to escalate, people started interrupting one another and tensions began to rise in the room. Sound familiar?
>
> I raised my hand and when called on said to the group, 'I see that everyone has something to contribute, so I'm wondering if we could try having this conversation in a different way. I'd like to suggest that we start at one end of the room and give everyone a chance to share what they believe we can do to salvage our time together given our circumstances. If you have nothing to add or if your idea has already been voiced, you may pass.'
>
> Everyone agreed and calm was restored; people no longer felt compelled to compete for air space. Each person shared their perspective and ideas began to build on the previous comments of others. After hearing from all 25 participants, the preferred solution became very apparent. Ultimately, we agreed to alter the two-day agenda and address all of the topics and activities that did not require technology at the front end of the summit, allowing for technical services to be put in place overnight and be ready for the group the following day. We also modified some of the strategies for delivering content to accommodate the limited internet access. While the solution was seemingly simple, it was a vast departure from where the conversation began. The resulting solution was a hybrid of several ideas and because everyone had a chance to contribute and hear the evolution of the thinking, we reached consensus and had broad support for the idea, rather than resignation and compliance.
>
> At the end of this round, one of the participants at the back of the room said, 'Wow that was amazing! I have never been in a room where people's ideas were treated with so much respect.' Our group reached a decision about an emotionally charged issue very quickly and respectfully. Everyone contributed and felt heard. Rather than competing to

champion individual ideas, the process of a round freed us up to listen to each person with full attention and arrive at a solution with the benefit of everyone's thinking.

Closing rounds are the last act of a *Positive and Productive Meeting*. They provide closure to the meeting and end everything on a positive, appreciative note. They can be used very effectively to help groups grow and deepen their practice of *Positive and Productive Meetings*.

Again, there is a standard closing round, as the principle here is to end the meeting with appreciation, using this question: 'What have you appreciated about our time together today/this meeting?'

AGENDA DEVELOPMENT

One of the best ways to focus conversation in a meeting and prevent it from being derailed is to create an agenda that helps people prepare for and organise meetings and reminds people why they meet.

Elements of a *Positive and Productive Meetings* agenda include:

Purpose: List your reason for meeting at the top of the agenda.

Logistics: Indicate the date, time and place of the meeting.

Roles: Write the names of team members who will be filling the meeting roles. There is no rule that the team leader or supervisor must facilitate all meetings. Mix it up. Assign different roles according to people's strengths and interests. If you use your agenda as your meeting minutes, include a space to list all in attendance.

Topic: What will the group be discussing during its time together? Items for information simply name the topic. Items for discussion are phrased as questions. This is a pivotal practice in *Positive and Productive Meetings*. If you think about meetings you have attended in the past, you are likely to have experienced agendas with one-word topics for discussion. Topics like 'budget', 'upcoming programmes' and 'staff participation' are all discussion items that are often seen listed on recent agendas.

These vague descriptors give little information about what is going to be discussed, what the group is hoping to accomplish or how participants can best prepare and contribute. As a result, members attending have to rely on their own assumptions about what the focus of the discussion is to be, because the agenda had not clearly defined the topic. Assumptions quickly lead us in many different directions, causing the discussion to evolve in circles and turn off into unrelated tangents.

For example, if you receive an agenda with a discussion item posted as 'staff participation', an immediate assumption may be that the group is going to discuss how to improve staff participation in your team meetings. Suddenly, you may find yourself thinking about all the problems and barriers to participation. The person to your left may have a totally different assumption about what this agenda topic means. It comes as no surprise that chaos and confusion are common outcomes for agenda items that are not clearly defined.

What if, instead, the agenda item is posed a question with a desired outcome, such as: 'What are some ways that we can recognise staff for their increased participation in meetings during this past quarter?' Our desired outcome is a list of possible strategies that will be forwarded to directors for review and approval.

This is suddenly a very different conversation about staff participation. You will know you are done with this agenda item when you have generated a list of ideas. The group is not being asked to decide and therefore do not need to invest extra time in advocating the merit of one strategy over another. If the desired outcome is a decision on the top two ideas, then you would know you probably need more time to consider the options and reach a decision.

Owner: The person who suggests an item for the agenda is usually the owner and will introduce the discussion during the meeting.

Decide or inform: Does the topic require the group's input, discussion and decision? Is the item just an update?

Desired outcome: What do you hope to accomplish by addressing this agenda item? Be specific, as this is a key tool in helping the group to stay on track.

Come prepared to: How should people prepare for this agenda item? This might include things to bring, materials to read or review in advance, and so on.

Time: How long is this agenda item expected to take?

Notes: Some groups record their meeting minutes directly onto the agenda, or use a reporting format based on the agenda. Meeting notes only need to document critical information, in particular any actions, issues or decisions.

> The Board of Directors of the Santa Ynez Valley Humane Society implemented *Positive and Productive Meetings* as part of a board development initiative. Kathy, the Executive Director, and Jody, Board President, were concerned that the board had got into the habit of having three-hour board meetings that resulted in few decisions and unclear outcomes. Members often left meetings exhausted and frustrated because they did not know what had been decided or who was supposed to do what.
>
> The entire board completed training in *Positive and Productive Meetings* and adopted these new agenda practices. After the training, Jody commented, 'Though usually I am not at a loss for words, all I can say right now is *wow*. What a great retreat, full of valuable information. I am so excited to implement the process. Who knew one could have so much to say about planning a meeting!'
>
> Kathy reported that by implementing the use of rounds and the new agenda format, the board cut their meeting time in half and more than doubled the number of decisions made during meetings; many board members commented on how much they appreciated hearing the perspectives of all participants. Kathy heard new ideas from board members that she had not expected, leading to more innovative solutions for the organisation.
>
> Figure 5.1 shows an example of one of their meeting agendas, using the *Positive and Productive Meetings* format.

Rounds and agenda development are two elements of a more comprehensive system of person-centred meeting practices. Figure 5.2 provides an overview of the process of conducting a *Positive and Productive Meeting.*

Agenda development: Everyone contributes their ideas for topics between meetings. People receive a copy of the agenda before the meeting starts.

Create a welcoming environment: People work best when they feel valued and are comfortable. Refreshments, lighting and seating are just a few things to consider.

Opening round: Start every meeting with an opening round. This helps people to stay connected and increases the likelihood that they will contribute during the meeting.

Review meeting map and assign roles: Check to make sure that everyone is clear on your meeting purpose and agenda items. Identify people who will help move the meeting forward. Clarify as needed.

Meeting maps have been called 'plans for meetings'. These are the foundation of meetings and provide a visual guide for the attendees. There are many ways to develop meeting maps. Some people use chart paper on the wall with graphics and colour, while others have all the information typed on letter-sized paper.

MEETING: SYVHS Board of Directors Meeting	DATE: Nov 21, 2011	TIME: 6:15 pm – 7:45 pm

ROLES:
Facilitator: Jody
Timekeeper: TBD
Recorder: TBD
Ground Rules Coach: Cheryl
Rounds Leader: TBD
Hospitality: TBD

STANDING ITEMS:

I.	**Purpose/Ground Rules**	2m
II.	**Opening Round:**	5m
III.	**Review Meeting Map**	4m
	a. Assign roles	
	b. Review rules	
	c. Review/revise agenda	
IV.	**Shelter Moment**	2m
V.	**Closing Round:**	5m
VI.	**Mission Statement**	2m

PURPOSE: The Santa Ynez Valley Humane Society Board of Directors ensures the fiscal viability, strategic direction and executive oversight of shelter programs and services, and educates the public of its mission to provide and promote humane, compassionate, and conscientious car e of companion animals and preventing their overpopulation.

MEETING GROUND RULES:
- Arrive on time
- Be respectful of the person leading the meeting
- Be prepared: read materials and bring to meeting
- Prioritize agenda items
- Demonstrate respect for person who has the floor
- Make decisions by majority vote

(90 minutes = 20 mins allocated to standing items; 70 mins for Discussion & Information Items)

VII. DISCUSSION ITEMS - Questions	Desired Outcome	Owner	Time	I/D	Come prepared to...
1. Purpose/Ground Rules	To review our board purpose and meeting ground rules	Cheryl	2 m	I	Listen
2. Opening Round: What is one positive thing you learned at our retreat?	Comments on retreat	RL	5 m	I	Make a comment about the retreat
3. Review Meeting Map a) Assign roles b) Review ground rules c) Review/revise agenda	Who will do what, and what we need to accomplish	Jody	4 m	D	Volunteer for roles
4. Shelter Moment	We hear a story about shelter services	Kathy	2 m	I	Listen
5. What suggestions do we have for handling tardiness to board meetings?	List of suggestions, to be referred to Strategic Committee (round)	Jody	10 m	D	Come with suggestion(s)
6. What types of events can board members suggest for the coming year (2012)?	List of suggestions (round, flip chart, end of meeting – dots), to be referred to Events Committee	Cheryl	30 m	D	Come with ideas for possible events for next year.

Figure 5.1 Extract from a meeting agenda in the Positive and Productive Meetings format

Summary of Positive and Productive meetings process

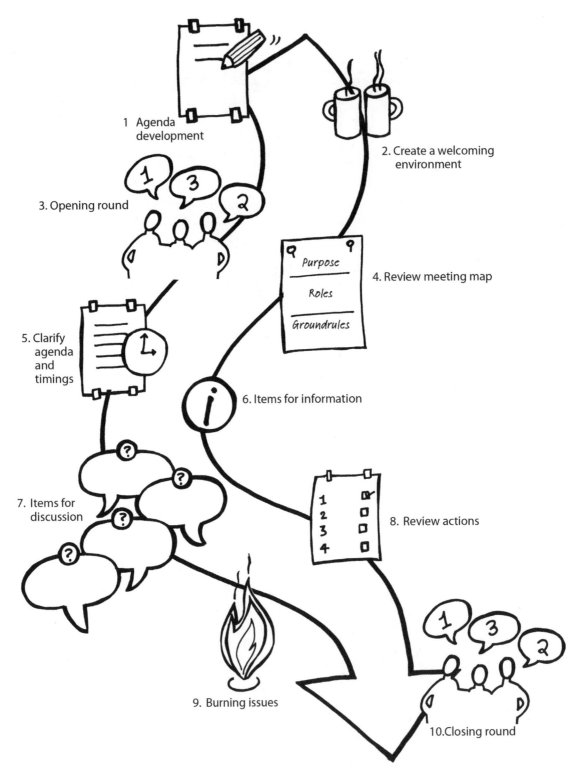

Figure 5.2 The process of a Positive and Productive Meeting

Review meeting groundrules (this is part of Review meeting Map): Ask participants what agreements can be established to ensure that the meeting remains positive and productive. Some sample agreements might include:

- Decisions are made with the majority vote of people at the meeting, unless the decision is to be made by the team leader.

- Cell phones are off or on vibrate and calls must be returned on breaks.

- We will have respectful discussions – one person talking at a time.

- Everyone should contribute in a way that is comfortable.

Clarify agenda and timings: Review the agenda and check the order, content and time for each item. Set realistic expectations and stick with them.

Items for information: Share updates and other informational agenda items. These items can be dispersed throughout the meeting to help balance your efforts.

Items for discussion: Creative ideas and collaborative problem solving are the great benefits of having group discussions on important agenda items.

Review actions: Confirm the group's to-do list before closing the meeting. This helps to build accountability and momentum. Write down who will do what, by when.

Burning issues: What didn't you have time for? What came up during the meeting that couldn't be addressed? Add these items to the next agenda, or determine the most appropriate course of action to address them further (i.e., delegate to a committee).

Closing round: End every meeting with a closing round. Having people share something they appreciated about the meeting helps to end on a positive note.

> Michelle Livesley and Cheryl Swan describe how they used *Positive and Productive Meetings* with colleagues in a hospital.
>
> Spiral Health began as a social enterprise on 1 April 2012. Prior to this, ward meetings were held on a monthly basis but there had been something of a lack of focus around meetings, and unclear objectives – when it came to meetings, people hadn't always felt able to contribute and there had been some conflict, with only sporadic attendance.
>
> Meeting agendas lacked real focus and were really more about giving information than engaging people in decision-making and discussion. Meetings were often very one-sided and when disagreement occurred it had the potential to result in a 'free-for-all'. It wasn't unknown for people to get quite emotional and leave feeling upset.
>
> But when the structure of the organisation changed, so did some of the personnel, and there was a real desire to do things differently.
>
> Spiral Health Managing Director Tracey Bush and Clinical Lead Cheryl Swan began considering what the best possible experience for staff and patients would be, and how meetings could contribute to this.
>
> Spiral were boosted by the previous experience that Tracey had of positive and productive meetings in other roles. She was using this in the meetings that she already chaired, such as workforce development, but she was keen to introduce it across all meetings in the organisation.
>
> Training was organised for all staff – regardless of job title or role, and it was seen as important that everyone learned and contributed to the development of Positive and *Productive Meetings* together. On day one of the training, the group came together to decide what the purpose of the ward meeting was – the group used a technique used in *Positive and Productive Meetings* called 'thinking rounds' to ensure that all views were considered, but it was difficult for the group to agree and it became clear that the purpose of the meeting was no longer understood.

It emerged that although meetings were much better than in the past, it was still felt that they were covering too much information, some of which didn't relate to the work taking place on the ward – and this was causing frustration. The group spent some time exploring what they wanted to achieve in the meeting, and used this discussion to clarify the purpose.

Once this had been clarified and recorded, it then became easy to figure out who should be attending, which items would need to be on the agenda and more importantly, which didn't. Jan Moutrey, the Nurse Lead, then took responsibility for taking the process forward and introducing it into the newly named 'clinical meetings'.

Following this, things have gone from strength to strength. People now share roles and responsibilities within the meeting, contribute to the agenda and are using thinking rounds to actively take part in meeting discussions. There's a much more collaborative atmosphere and people are feeling positive and motivated when leaving the meeting.

The staff coming together to contribute to the agenda has made a huge difference to overall understanding of the meeting's purpose, and the meetings have become more positive and productive as a result.

Practice clear, shared decision making

Every day people make decisions that affect other people. Person-centred teams create clarity about how decisions are made and how people are listened to, consulted or informed about decisions.

While it is not always practical or possible to have every person who could be affected by a decision present and involved at all times, person-centred teams honour a facilitative and participative leadership approach.[44]

Despite the merits of increasing participation in decision making, people may fear a loss of control over the outcome or the process of getting there, or they may think that their way of doing things is the best or quickest.

The key to increasing involvement without losing control is to seek the maximum involvement *appropriate* to the situation. When making decisions as a team leader, first think about all the key decisions you might make for the team, then consider the following questions:

- What decisions do you make on your own?
- What decisions do team members make on their own?
- What decisions do the entire team need to be involved in making?
- What decisions do you consult with others on, even though you make the final decision?

Another approach that's particularly useful when working with other agencies is to consider which decisions:

- are yours to make
- are theirs to make
- are made together.

> Jennie is a young woman who lives in a flat supported by a team of staff from a local provider organisation. Her mum, Suzie, has a circle of support of friends and family (a team in the context of this book) to support her make sure that Jennie has the best life possible. As Jennie has autism and does not have the legal capacity to employ her own staff, Suzie and the circle do this on her behalf, and employ the provider to support Jennie. It has been very successful overall, but occasionally there are tensions over decision making.

Recently, the manager changed the shift pattern of the staff, and the circle felt that this should have been a decision that they made together.

The circle used the simplified decision-making agreement to start the discussion with the provider about where decisions needed to be made together.

Table 5.2 Decision making about Jennie's life and service

What is yours? (decisions the provider makes by themselves)	What is ours? (decisions the circle makes themselves)	What decisions need to be shared? (that we have to make or agree on together)
What happens in supervision sessions with the team leader?	How often, when and where the circle meets.	Changes to the shift pattern.

Who needs to be involved in decision making?

When considering who needs to be involved in a decision, or who can help with a decision, it is beneficial to think broadly about those who are affected. A person who is affected by a decision who may be able to help is anyone (or group of people) who:

- is responsible for making the final decision

- is in a position to carry out the decision or prevent it from being implemented

- is likely to be affected by the outcome of the decision

- has information or expertise related to the decision.

One way to answer the question 'Who can help?' is to use a relationship circle (see Figure 5.3). First, identify who could be affected by the decision. Place their names on the relationship circle according to your comfort level and confidence in working with them. The names closest to the centre represent people with whom you have a good rapport. Names on the outer circle might be people with whom you have a more distant personal connection.

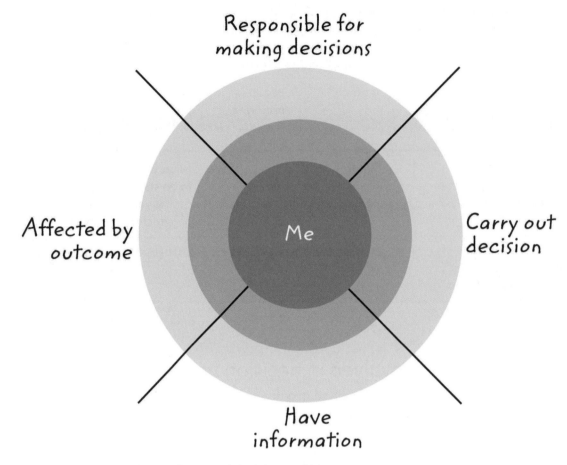

Figure 5.3 A relationship circle around decision making

HOW ARE YOU AND OTHERS INVOLVED IN THE DECISION?

Think about different ways people can make decisions and carry them out. An acronym that can clarify maximum engagement and empowerment is RASIC,[45] a model commonly used in project management literature that stands for:

R   **Responsible:** A person or group that recommends a decision.

A   **Approve:** The person or group that approves the decision.

S   **Support:** Anyone who has a role in the decision's implementation.

I   **Inform:** People who are kept up to date on progress; one-way communication.

C   **Consult:** People whose opinions are sought, and with whom there is two-way communication.

In this variation of a decision-making agreement, RASIC is used to identify clearly who is involved in a decision and what role they play.

Table 5.3 *Using RASIC to identify roles*

How will we mitigate the negative impact of budget cuts on direct services?					
Who can help?	Directors	Staff	People receiving support	Service providers	Funders
How can they help?	A	R, C, S	C	C, S	I, S

This brief example shows how one social care agency looked at all of the people involved in a decision and sorted out who needed to be consulted, informed and notified of the decision. This decision-making matrix helped them to plan their course of action on an important topic affecting many people. This can be a useful clarifying tool for planning teams and circles of support.

Process question 2: how will we achieve success?

To look at the second success question, let's go back to the emerging one-page strategy for the training team Housing Associates that we started in Chapter 2. Here you can see that delivering success really depends on what the team's business is. You would expect to see current thinking on excellence in learning and development in relation to how this training team delivers success. However, where success for the team includes members supporting each other and being clear about expectations, you can see some of the processes we have mentioned included. Table 5.4 shows the processes that they decided to use to achieve their success statements:

Table 5.4 *Processes in achieving success*

Success from different perspectives			
Participants	Customers	Team	Organisation
Participants have new skills they can use in their workplace. Participants have new knowledge that's useful to them in their workplace. The training is engaging and builds on participants' existing knowledge.	The training achieves outcomes in an efficient and engaging manner.	We feel supported. We learn together and continually improve our service.	Training is delivered to customers' satisfaction in a way that reflects our values and is within budget.

cont.

Participants	Customers	Team	Organisation
How will we deliver success?			
Use engaging blended learning approaches (e-learning, webinars, etc.) as well as face-to-face training. Use survey monkeys to establish how much people know and what skills they have, and design the training around this to build on existing skills and knowledge. Involve potential participants in designing new learning experiences.	Know how far we can go in delivering our customers' outcomes (team Doughnut)? Create a one-page summary for each customer that shows how we plan to deliver their outcomes. A bespoke short report for each customer on how we delivered their outcomes, with quotes from participants and scores from survey monkey.	All team members have a one-page profile so we know how to support each other. We use *Positive and Productive Meetings*. We use person-centred supervision to reflect on learning and to problem solve. We have a person-centred team plan that describes how we work together.	Review the budget together in individual supervision sessions, and every quarter during team meetings.
How will we know we're successful?			
The percentage of participants who score 70 per cent or more in our course follow-up evaluation (survey monkey) that state they have new skills and knowledge they can use in their workplace. The percentage of participants who score 70 per cent or more in relation to the training being engaging.	In our post-course evaluation the percentage of customers who rate us good or excellent in response to the statement: 'The training achieved our outcomes.'	We review the support section in our one-page profile with our manager every quarter and develop actions based on what is working and not working. We have an annual whole-team person-centred review and agree on actions from this.	Delivering our service within budget.

Teams who are focused on delivering personalised support to people in health, education and care will also be using person-centred practices in how they deliver success.

The team working to deliver personalised support to people living with dementia at Bruce Lodge developed the following strategy in Figure 5.4. You can see how person-centred practices, in particular one-page profiles and person-centred reviews, were central to delivering success.

Personalising Care Homes
One-Page Strategy

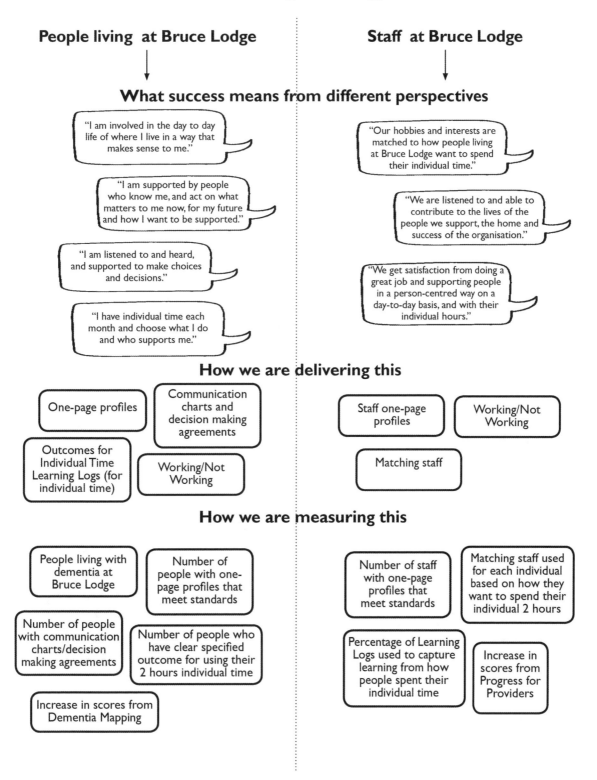

People living at Bruce Lodge

Staff at Bruce Lodge

What success means from different perspectives

"I am involved in the day to day life of where I live in a way that makes sense to me."

"I am supported by people who know me, and act on what matters to me now, for my future and how I want to be supported."

"I am listened to and heard, and supported to make choices and decisions."

"I have individual time each month and choose what I do and who supports me."

"Our hobbies and interests are matched to how people living at Bruce Lodge want to spend their individual time."

"We are listened to and able to contribute to the lives of the people we support, the home and success of the organisation."

"We get satisfaction from doing a great job and supporting people in a person-centred way on a day-to-day basis, and with their individual hours."

How we are delivering this

One-page profiles

Communication charts and decision making agreements

Outcomes for Individual Time Learning Logs (for individual time)

Working/Not Working

Staff one-page profiles

Working/Not Working

Matching staff

How we are measuring this

People living with dementia at Bruce Lodge

Number of people with one-page profiles that meet standards

Number of people with communication charts/decision making agreements

Number of people who have clear specified outcome for using their 2 hours individual time

Increase in scores from Dementia Mapping

Number of staff with one-page profiles that meet standards

Matching staff used for each individual based on how they want to spend their individual 2 hours

Percentage of Learning Logs used to capture learning from how people spent their individual time

Increase in scores from Progress for Providers

Figure 5.4 Extract from the one-page strategy for My Home, My Life, My Choice

★

Steps to Success

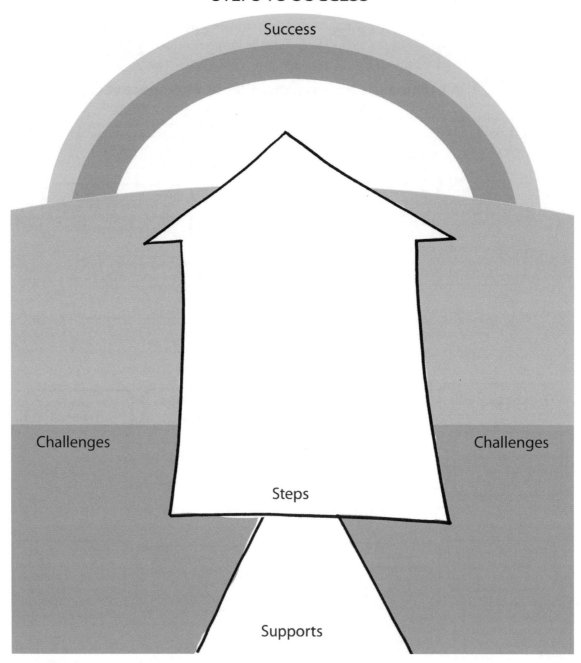

Figure 5.5 Steps to Success graphic template

For many teams, achieving success requires specific steps that need to be turned into goals and actions. We are covering this here, as it is a process to achieve success. Goals will are also generated from a review of progress (which we cover in the next chapter). One simple planning process to move a team towards their definition of success is called *Steps to Success*.

As you can see, the template is a simple way to record what success looks like and the actions a team need to take to move towards that success. It includes a place to record barriers and opportunities addressed within the action planning. The case study below gives an example of how one team used a graphic template.

> The leadership team of a national provider was exploring how they could ensure their services were as person-centred and personalised as possible. They started with the question: *'If we were very successful in delivering truly personalised services, what would this look and feel like for the people we support, the staff and the organisation?'*
>
> Individually they thought about the question and wrote their ideas on coloured cards. They paired with other team members and shared the cards to find consensus and differences. Then they clustered the cards into themes and labelled them in three categories:
>
> - People we support will choose their own staff.
>
> - The morale in the organisation will be high.
>
> - Staff will know exactly what is expected of them and where they can use their own judgement.
>
> They put each of the success statements on the *Steps to Success* poster. For each statement the group thought about how they would know if they had achieved that success (i.e., staff morale and satisfaction are measured through an annual questionnaire). Once the group agreed on how they would measure success, they thought about the opportunities and barriers to achieving that success and ended with five bold action steps.

Steps to Success is a useful tool to ensure that actions are in place to move the entire team towards performance statements. Successful person-centred teams would review the template and their actions at team meetings. As well as this happening together as a team, there needs to be opportunities to reflect together at an individual level.

An important process for ensuring that team members stay focused on delivering performance, work within team agreements and have opportunities to problem solve and acknowledge learning and success is one-to-one sessions with the team leader.

MATCHING

One-page strategies summarise the most important ways a team can deliver performance. *Steps to Success* is useful when the team needs to think differently about how it's working to deliver success and implement a plan to develop new ways of working or to make changes. The next decision is who is the best person to deliver on key tasks, or to be matched to roles, customers or people who utilise the company's services.

How to get the best fit between individual team members and the work that has to be done will be one of the most important decisions you'll make as a team leader. There are different ways to discover your staff's strengths:

- There will be clues in their one-page profile (i.e., the appreciation section will show areas of strength). People tend to enjoy what they're best at, so look at what they say is important in their work. People are more likely to need help in areas where they lack talent, so the support section can provide clues.

- Use the Strengths Finder developed by Marcus Buckingham.[46]

- Use personality tests such as Myers-Briggs Type Indicator (MBTI).

If you use any of these tools, make sure the information is added to one-page profiles.

In a person-centred team we go beyond just working to people's strengths – we try to look at shared common interests as well. The Learning Community for Person-Centred Practices developed the 'matching tool' as a way to help get this match right. This includes sections on the support that the person needs, the skills needed to support that person, the ideal personality characteristics of the people involved and, where possible, the interests it would be good for people to share.

United Response is developing a person-centred service supporting people with dementia who live at home. Hilda was the first person to use this service. Nick, a manager with United Response, met with Hilda and her niece Gill to develop a one-page profile for Hilda, which could be used as a basis for deciding on the best staff to support her. He used the matching tool.

These are Helen's observations of that meeting:

> As I left the meeting last night Hilda and Nick were comparing notes about old movies they loved. Hilda was discussing her all-time favourite with Cary Grant, talking knowledgeably about the original involving the Empire State Building, and the remake set in the plane.
>
> Nick and I had met Hilda for the first time with her niece, Gill, to begin the process of delivering person-centred home care to Hilda. Hilda calls this her 'personal shopper'. Hilda is 92, a fantastic film buff; she lives by herself near the coast, is registered blind and now is in the early stages of dementia.
>
> Gill and her daughters, Barbara and Rachel, support Hilda and stay over a couple of nights a week. She has great neighbours, too, Jean and Brian, who call in every day. Her daughter, Joan, lives in the States in Pittsburgh, and while we were there Joan phoned Hilda to see how the meeting was going.
>
> For Gill and Joan and for Hilda too, there had been one too many near misses with traffic as Hilda crossed roads on the way to the shops. She also needed more and more help to find the items she required and to read her shopping list as her eyesight was deteriorating.
>
> Nick and I met with Gill and Hilda for an hour to learn about her and what she wanted from a service. Here is some of what I learned about Hilda through purposeful conversation and from being introduced to her family through the array of precious photographs in the lounge and kitchen:

> - She goes shopping every Sunday with Gill to Clevelys, where they have lunch in the café and Hilda buys a new film on DVD.
>
> - She is a great cook – while we were there she talked about the scones she was planning to make.
>
> - She loves watching soaps as well as her old films, in particular her favourites are *Emmerdale* and *Strictly Come Dancing*. She enjoys getting the answers right when she watches *Eggheads*.
>
> - Her garden is important to her – it has raised beds, and Hilda makes new hanging baskets each spring.
>
> - Her family is central to her life – seeing Barbara and Rachel, and speaking to Joan and the family in the States each week, on a Sunday and a Tuesday at 5pm.

> I learned about what people love and admire about Hilda from talking to Gill when we were arranging the first meeting. Hilda has a great sense of fun, is incredibly organised and tells it like it is!

From this meeting there was enough information to develop Hilda's profile and complete the matching tool, which is how United Response learned about what Hilda was looking for from staff. Nick's task was to look at the one-page profiles he had for his staff who lived in the same neighbourhood as Hilda, and see who the best match was for her. It became clear after assessing the profiles that Linda was the best match.

Table 5.5 Matching Support to Hilda

Support needed.	• Support with shopping and paying the paper bill. • Minimal support getting in and out of the car. • Link arms while walking.
Skills needed.	• Good conversationalist. • Car driver.
Personality characteristics needed.	• Ideally a mature woman. • Outgoing without being loud. • At ease with people. • Sensitive. • Confident. • Empathetic.
Shared interests if possible.	• Old movies and movie stars. • Music such as Vera Lynn, Susan Boyle, Aled Jones and singers from the 1940s and 1950s.

Now you have ways to explore working together and meeting as a team. We've also discussed specific ways of working that will enable you to deliver success (perhaps described in your one-page strategy). During this journey of discovery you may have thought about additional changes you'll need to make to achieve success (i.e., using processes like *Steps to Success*), and how to get the best match between your team and their required tasks and roles using the matching tool.

Next you need to consider how you can support your team in delivering thorough one-to-one sessions. These are given a range of names from supervision, job consultation, appraisals or one-to-ones. But we prefer *supervision*, and in the next section we describe what a person-centred approach could look like.

Adopt a person-centred approach to supervision

Supervision meetings can be experienced by staff as a negative, almost punitive, experience. This person-centred approach to supervision focuses on opportunities for appreciation and feedback, reflection on progress and learning, and an opportunity for shared problem solving.

Here, one-page profiles are very important. In supervision, the staff member and manager can look at team purpose and performance expectations and think about what support the staff member will need to deliver them (and ensure they get the support described in their one-page profile). When an issue arises in supervision, at the end of the session the manager and staff member can discuss what they learned about the person or the support they need that should be added to or changed on their one-page profile.

Innovative organisations use staff one-page profiles within supervision to find out what is/isn't working from the staff member and their manager's perspective, then agree on actions that build on what is working and address what is not working.

Carolynn

Carolynn, a manager, was trained by Michelle to use a person-centred approach, and this is how it changed her thinking and methods of practice.

Carolynn believed that staff had a historical perception of supervision being punitive, and therefore it was a negative experience, regardless of how she had tried to approach it. Staff saw supervision as a time to be 'told off' and therefore there was reluctance to attend and contribute.

Carolynn said that the meetings were often one-sided, with her deciding on the majority of the agenda. She made up for this by making sure lots of informal, unplanned support was given with an open-door type of philosophy; because of this, there was a tendency for structured supervisions to be infrequent, although informal guidance was available at any time.

The point of staff supervision is to allow for time and space to focus on supporting staff through the structural and ideological changes taking place, and on the outcomes for the individuals being supported. Staff needed to understand their roles within the changes, and that the one-to-one time afforded by supervision ensured that there were opportunities for reflection.

Michelle had a session with Carolynn that equipped her with a person-centred process to help her to support her staff team more effectively. They explored how the content of supervision should have a focus on what they were learning about the team and the people they support, and how they were progressing with the outcomes developed via the support planning and subsequent planning opportunities.

Carolynn said that she felt more confident to support staff by using the supervision process and that the structure had really helped her to have more meaningful conversations with them.

She now realises that before this process of change, supervision of her staff and other people she supported was not always 100 per cent person-centred, despite aiming for it to be so. Originally, staff meetings focused on policy and procedures, because that's what staff were most concerned about.

This support focused on Carolynn's management style, and made her feel as though she was putting efforts forth in a more productive and fruitful way. For Carolynn, 'Being able to ask my staff what they wanted from supervision, and moving away from the negative associations of staff supervision, is great!'

The NHS Employers organisation issued some key tips for employers during their rounds of appraisal and objective setting that included:[47]

- Be patient focused.

- Ensure that individual objectives link to your organisation's objectives.

- Foster a culture of performance management in your team.

These points suggest that a stronger focus may be required for some employers around being person- or patient-centred and reviewing objectives and performance. Following a process that is person-centred enables team leaders to focus on performance and objectives.

Person-centred supervision enables team leaders to encourage staff to deliver performance standards and to make sure that they clearly understand what is expected of them.

Summary of person-centred supervision (one-to-ones)

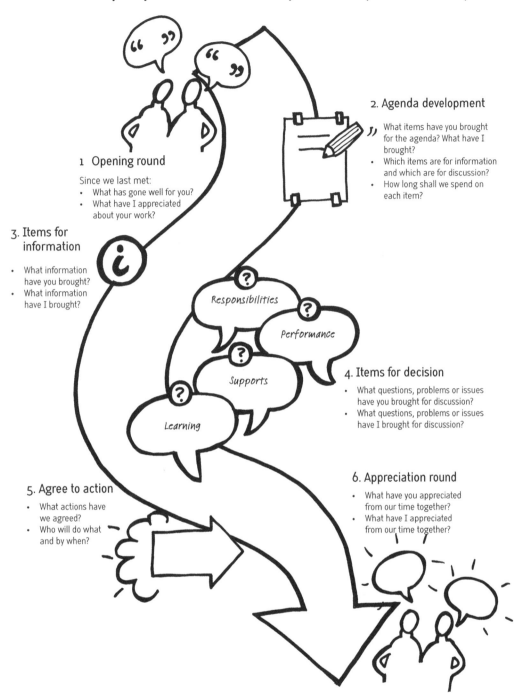

Figure 5.6 The process of person-centred supervision

Maureen

Maureen loves technology, and is very creative in using visual imagery, video and sound in PowerPoint to design engaging learning modules. She understands eLearning technology better than most other team members.

She shared that one of her aspirations is to eventually be an instructional design consultant. Because of her interests and expertise, she agreed to serve as project coordinator for a statewide eLearning development initiative. As a result of that assignment, a list of tasks, responsibilities and success indicators were created to help her be successful in her new role. Their task statement included:

• Developing 15 eLearning modules on topics determined by chief counsellors to serve as a statewide core curriculum that provided greater consistency for new service co-ordinator orientation.

• Developing modules that adhered to eLearning practice standards that were to be editable by each regional centre and delivered via a statewide learning management system by 31 May.

The task statement included three major elements for developing clear and compelling performance goals:

• Action (develop eLearning modules).

• Why it's important to serve as a statewide core curriculum that provides greater consistency.

• What it looks like when done well.

The group developed a shared Doughnut to clarify the expectations and alignment between the organisation, the Training and Information Group, and Maureen.

Table 5.6 *Using person-centred supervision with Maureen*

Co-ordinator Orientation eLearning initiative	Core responsibility	Creativity and judgement	Beyond our responsibility
Organisation: Statewide Association.	Convene one of the standing committees to implement this priority. Identify the core learning titles and topics to be included in the training modules. Approve funding to provide a statewide learning management system (LMS) that will be the vehicle for delivering the online learning modules.	Looking at different strategies for funding the purchase of a statewide LMS.	Whether or not all member agencies choose to participate in the shared purchase of an LMS.
Team: Training Committee.	Reach an agreement on core learning objectives to be included in the training modules. Define instructional design standards to develop shared content. Research and propose LMS vendor for executive directors' approval. Develop a plan to roll out and administer the statewide LMS.	What types of instructional interactions will be used. Whether the module will be created in Articulate or Captivate.	Introducing other statewide content without director approval. Whether or not all member agencies choose to participate in the shared purchase of an LMS.
Individual: Maureen.	Provide quarterly updates to TIG on status of LMS implementation. Serve as liaison between Training Committee and the LMS vendor.	Methods of delivering instructional support for system administrators.	Ensuring that each member agency successfully launches and implements the core curriculum.

If you were Maureen's team manager how might you use person-centred supervision to support her in achieving these performance standards? Table 5.6 provides an example of how your supervision could be structured.

Opening round: How would you appreciate Maureen in the opening round? Perhaps something about the creativity she brings to her work? Maureen would then mention what she appreciates about the support you're giving her.

Agenda Development: This session would focus on performance, learning and support. Maureen may suggest the order she would find most useful.

Items for Discussion or Decision

Learning: What has Maureen learned through working on the project? You might use the *four-plus-one questions* to help structure this:

1. What have you tried?

2. What have you learned?

3. What are you pleased about?

4. What are you concerned about?

Based on the answers to these questions, what could she do next? It is to be hoped that Maureen learned about herself and the support she needs through this experience, so you could encourage her to update her profile with this information.

Performance: You could talk to Maureen about what is/isn't working in delivering on the performance standards from your perspective – look at each one in relation to her development and liaison role, and provide quarterly updates.

This is where issues around competency would be addressed. Are there any new competencies Maureen requires to do her tasks brilliantly? What learning opportunities and support would this require? How would you know if this was making a difference to her skill set and knowledge?

Support: You'll want to ask Maureen if she felt supported by other team members and by you as her manager. You might ask her 'What would excellent support look like?' and 'What could be done to make it happen?' (there may be valuable information to add to the support section in her one-page profile). You could negotiate what would be realistic yet supportive, and suggest she starts to develop more comprehensive *stress and support* information.

Appreciations: At the end of the session you could tell Maureen what you appreciated about her contribution during your one-to-one session, and encourage her to do the same.

Getting started

How you work together as a team has huge breadth in terms of issues to consider and ideas to explore. There are likely to be some areas you feel pleased about and proud of how you are doing, and other areas that you want to improve and develop. Are there more productive ways to use everyone's time? Do you make decisions and see results from your meetings? Does everyone share responsibility for making them a success? Our recommendation would be to start with meetings if your answer to any of these questions is no. Here are some suggestions about how to get started.

WHAT DO YOU THINK YOUR TEAM NEEDS?

The bottom line is that you, as the team leader, need to feel confident that your team can and will deliver on its performance expectations. What would that take? What are the actions to take – for example, *Steps to Success*, or working with individuals to help them deliver?

HEAR WHAT EVERYONE'S TOP PRIORITIES ARE

Although we would suggest starting with meetings, it is up to you and your team to decide on your priorities. You could simply ask team members what they think is working and not working about how you work together as a team and deliver your purpose. Another possibility is to ask each person if they could change one thing about how the team works together, what would that be?

When Miguel asked his fellow support worker, Marcella, this question, she said, 'For everyone to take their fair share in keeping the house clean.' Marcella supported three people with learning disabilities in a group home. Miguel thought that this simple answer told him a lot. It suggested that:

- success for Marcella included how clean and tidy the house is, and this does not feature at all in the team's success statements, so he needed to find out how important (or not) this was to the whole team

- there were issues in how tasks were allocated and shared within the team.

As a result of this (and other team members' answers) the team spent time revisiting their success statements, looking at how roles and responsibilities were allocated within the team, and how decisions were made. This resulted in the team agreeing whole-team ground rules, and making sure these were reviewed every two months.

MAKE SURE MEETINGS ARE POSITIVE AND PRODUCTIVE

You can use the same questions in a team meeting: 'What is or isn't working?' and 'If you could change one thing, what would it be?' Sometimes team members may have very low expectations due to previous or existing experiences; or their managers might decide to introduce new ideas to the team and then evaluate them after a designated period of time so that the team can decide what to keep or discard.

It's relatively easy to introduce rounds at the beginning of meetings. When the team becomes used to the idea of an uninterrupted round, you can bring them in during different points on the agenda and at the end during the recap session. Alternatively, you can spend the day looking at all the tools and processes in *Positive and Productive Meetings* and vote on the ones to use.

CHANGE SUPERVISION TO MAKE IT MORE PERSON-CENTRED

As team leader you can change your supervision and one-to-one or appraisal practices, and use everyone's one-page profile in review sessions. And you can add information about performance to the emerging person-centred team plan.

Recording process in the person-centred team plan

By now we are hoping that you have some of the basic components of a team plan, for example:

- A clear description of your team's purpose, what success looks like and how you will know how successful you are. This could be a one-page strategy.

- Information about the people in your team – each person's one-page profile.

- You might have more detailed information about expectations – for example, a team Doughnut – and you might also have a synthesis of what is important to your team, and how best to support your team, taken from all of your one-page profiles.

Here are some ideas about how you can integrate your decisions about the processes your team will use in the team plan.

START WITH GUIDELINES OR GROUND RULES

Now you want to add information about how you work together. This could be team guidelines or ground rules.

Figure 5.7 shows the ground rules the Oxnard Children's Team added to this section of their team plan.

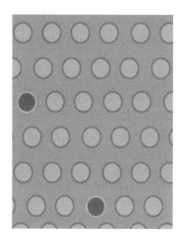

GROUND RULES
Listen to each other
Respect each other
Be safe
Relax
Cell phones on vibrate
Have fun, laugh

Figure 5.7 Ground Rules for the Oxnard Children's Team

ADD DETAILS

This can be the beginning of more detailed agreements about how your team works together. This could include information about meetings, supervision and conflict. Here are some examples:

Our development team meets for half a day every month. Everyone attends each meeting unless they are away from work (on leave or sick). We start and finish our meetings on time so please do not book appointments close to the beginning of the meeting that would cause a problem for you to be there on time.

We encourage people to talk directly and openly when we are upset with someone in the team. If we talk to someone else about being upset with another team member, then this person offers three approaches to dealing with it:

- Support the person to talk to the team member they are upset with.

- Offer to go with the person to do this.

- Offer to tell the person themselves.

Obviously the first two are better than the last, but the bottom line is that we must not harbour frustrations or be upset with each other. If it is upsetting enough to talk to someone else about, then that person shares a responsibility to make sure the issue is resolved with the person concerned.

GET THE RIGHT BALANCE BETWEEN RULES AND PRINCIPLES

Earlier we looked at the importance of moving away from rules to focus on principles. To reflect that, one team went from clear statements about what clothing was appropriate (for example, never to wear denim or combat trousers) to 'dress in a way that reflects our brand – professional and creative'. This team leader went even further to enable team members to think what this meant for them. She organised a day with a colour consultant so that each team member (men and women) could think about the impact of their colour and style choices and the impression that they made on customers.

Your person-centred team plan will be growing by now, as you think with your team about how you can work together to deliver success. All the building blocks are in place for your team to deliver excellence.

The next chapter is Progress, which teaches your staff how to be a team that's continually developing and learning and improving what they do.

Table 5.7 Process checklist

Process checklist	Strongly disagree	Disagree	Agree	Strongly agree
I understand formal and informal team rules.	☐	☐	☐	☐
I know how to use *Positive and Productive Meetings* practices, including rounds and agenda development.	☐	☐	☐	☐
I know how to make my supervision more person-centred.	☐	☐	☐	☐
I know how decisions are made in our team.	☐	☐	☐	☐
I consider different perspectives when handling conflict.	☐	☐	☐	☐
I know how to add process information to a team plan.	☐	☐	☐	☐

Chapter 6

Progress

The most viable organisations are the ones that understand that taking time to learn is never a waste of time.

Jeanne M. Plas[48]

Jim Collins said, 'The main thing is to keep the main thing the main thing.'[49] Checking progress helps to do just that.

The next part of a person-centred team is progress, where we'll discuss elements of continuous improvement and a learning culture. This isn't the last part of developing a person-centred team; quite the contrary, since progress is the loop back to the other sections.

Progress is where people learn how they are doing and what they can improve. They'll learn more about each other (people), set higher standards for themselves (performance), or adapt processes on the basis of what they are learning (processes).

Progress therefore is the hub of learning and improvement and ensures that the other Ps in person-centred teams are developed and updated. Although progress is critically important, it's often overlooked, under-utilised, and seen as an after-thought.

In this chapter we discuss the importance of focusing on progress, and suggest person-centred practices to explore the following questions:

- How are we doing?

- How can we improve?

For each of these questions, the answers will need to be explored from an individual and team perspective about how the team works together to deliver results.

Finally, we need to consider the interface between team and organisational learning. Here we'll focus on key person-centred practices, which you can position alongside existing ways to review progress and improve the team, such as satisfaction questionnaires, dashboards, 360-degree appraisals, action learning sets, etc.

In the previous chapter we looked at how to know how well you're doing as a team. In this chapter we'll give you more ideas and processes to add to that information.

Table 6.1 Addressing the progress questions

Progress question	You will have finished this section when...	Person-centred practices that can help
How are we doing?	*Individually* You review how supported individuals feel to deliver at their best, and how they feel around their well-being.	Learning log. What's working/not working around one-page profiles.
	You have a way of evaluating your individual performance.	Four-plus-one questions. Five Ways to Well-Being.
	As a team You review how well the team is working together.	Person-centred supervision. Person-centred team review.
	You review how the team is performing in relation to success.	Four-plus-one questions. Working Together for Change
How can we improve?	*Individually* You know how you can coach and support staff to improve.	To GROW. Four-plus-one questions.
	As a team You know how to problem solve what is getting in the way of improvements and come up with new ideas.	Working Together for Change.

Why is progress important?

In the Performance chapter we defined what you need to do to deliver purpose and clarify the results. In the Process chapter you learned how to deliver success, and in this chapter you'll learn ways to see how far you've progressed.

Progress refers to creating opportunities to learn from successes, challenges and even the most disappointing failures. Insights and lessons learned can redirect actions to keep us moving towards the intended target (an essential practice of a person-centred team). Many teams struggle to identify meaningful measures of success, and even fewer have a consistent way to monitor, discuss and report on progress.

Monitoring progress and building transparency about results can be a motivator to strive for excellence, and can engage team members in new and exciting ways that lead to greater productivity and positive results.

What does 'progress' mean?

Person-centred practices are used to check progress towards individual performance objectives, team effectiveness objectives, and many teams have project outcomes too. When members of a person-centred team check their progress they deliberately:

- seek input from multiple perspectives

- use their person-centred team plan to frame learning and problem solving

- learn from successes, challenges and failures, and use those insights to make informed decisions about the next steps.

Reflection on progress is powerful when it is done on a daily basis by individual team members, through person-centred practices such as *learning logs,* monthly review meetings using the *four-plus-one questions,* or annually through person-centred reviews. We explain each of these in this chapter.

SEEK INPUT FROM MULTIPLE PERSPECTIVES

In the same way that we explored purpose and success from different perspectives, stakeholders' views need to be taken into consideration when exploring progress. This can happen for individual staff members through established practices like 360-degree reviews.

In person-centred teams we look at the entire scope of progress in relation to people and families the team supports via person-centred reviews, and as a whole team through *Working Together for Change.*

USE THE TEAM PLAN TO FRAME LEARNING AND PROBLEM SOLVING

Using your person-centred team plan as a guide, periodically check on your plan to evaluate your progress but don't stop with just performance.

Because progress is, in part, about being accountable for results, teams that do check progress focus primarily on their performance indicators, contract deliverables and outcomes. Focusing only on results, and possibly overlooking the needs of team members and how the work gets done, makes it difficult to sustain excellent results over time.

Lasting success requires attention to relationships and process, and balanced attention to the five elements of a person-centred team: purpose, people, performance, process and progress.

Learn from successes, challenges and failures, and use the insights to inform decisions about next steps.

Teams that have a healthy learning culture reflect on an experience, consider the significance of that experience and determine what will be done next as a result of the experience.

Teams often go from reflecting on an experience to determining the next steps without considering the significance. The act of considering the *significance* of the experience is where insight and wisdom are born.

Ask yourself what is important about this experience? What has the team learned and how can that help in other situations? After reflecting on those questions, think about what the next steps will be.

In this section we are going to look at the first progress question – how are we doing, at an individual and a team level. Some of the processes we suggest for this have already been covered earlier in the book and we will point you to these.

Progress question 1: how are we doing?

When you talk to individual team members about how they are doing, this could be about their performance, how they are doing as part of the team, and their general well-being. Each of these is most likely to take place during one-to-one or supervision sessions, although some of these suggestions can also be adapted to use within team meetings. The person-centred practices that we find the most useful here are *learning logs, four-plus-one questions, working and not working* from different perspectives, and the *Five Ways to Well-Being*.

LEARNING LOGS

A *learning log* is a simple way for team members to record what they are learning about a particular event or how they are supporting someone. Many health and social care organisations require staff to complete progress notes in order to describe what happened. A *learning log* differs from progress notes as it not only records what happened, but what staff have learned and what they need to do differently next time.

John is living with dementia and his home for the last three years has been an independent hospital in the north west of England. John is a retired landscape gardener, he has been married to his wife Nell for 45 years and he has a daughter Lisa. The team who support John were aware that he rarely moved out of the lounge in the hospital and no longer used any words to speak. They decided to explore trying new activities with John, and used *learning logs* to record how he reacted and what they learned. Figure 6.1 is an example of one of the *learning logs*.

From the *learning log* it is clear that John loves the outdoors, and they now take every opportunity to support him to spend time at garden centres and in parks. John's family think that this has made a big difference to his well-being.

FOUR-PLUS-ONE QUESTIONS

This is a powerful person-centred thinking tool to help staff reflect on their progress and what they learned. It's comprised of four questions for information-gathering, plus one question for creating action steps. The questions that collect information help people consider different perspectives before moving to action.

In person-centred supervision, the *four-plus-one questions* support team members to reflect on how they did in delivering personal objectives. (We suggested how this could look for Maureen in the Process chapter.)

A national charity supporting people with long-term conditions meet monthly with an individual and their key worker to look at the previous month's progress, and use the *four-plus-one questions* to identify what they want to do differently the following month. The key worker's manager reviews this with them during their supervision session.

USING WORKING/NOT WORKING FROM DIFFERENT PERSPECTIVES

Working/not working from different perspectives is a way to reflect on what is going well and what needs to change. This can be done with individual team members around their performance, and in relation to their one-page profile. The process starts with the one-page profile and would usually take place during a supervision or appraisal meeting.

Beforehand, the team leader and the staff member prepare by both writing what they think is working and not working:

- in relation to the staff member and their performance

- in relation to the staff member's one-page profile (paying particular attention to how they want to be supported at work).

Learning Log

Date	Time	What did the person do? (what, where, when, how long, etc.)	Who was there? (Names of staff, friends, others, etc.)	What did you learn about what worked well? What did the person like about the activity? What needs to stay the same?
10th September	11.00am – 2.30pm	John went to the Trafford Centre to go shopping for some new clothes.	Sam (a member of staff), and Bill (who lives at the hospital).	John enjoyed lunch in pizza hut – ham and pineapple pizza. He took great interest in the plants and flowers section in Marks and Spencers.
17th September	2.00pm – 3.00pm	John went to a pottery class in the hospital.	Michelle (support staff), Jess the craft instructor, Tom and Nora (who live with him).	Standing at the window looking outdoors whistling when he heard the birds singing - his eyes lit up.
23th September	11.00am – 12 noon	John went out into the garden.	Pat (staff member)	John showed enjoyment whilst sweeping up the autumn leaves – humming and general feel he was engaged and content, loved feeling the leaves in his hands. Listening to the birds and rubbing his hand along the bark of the trees, Pat's knowledge of plants and their Latin names was of great benefit – John seemed to listen intently.

Figure 6.1 Learning log for John

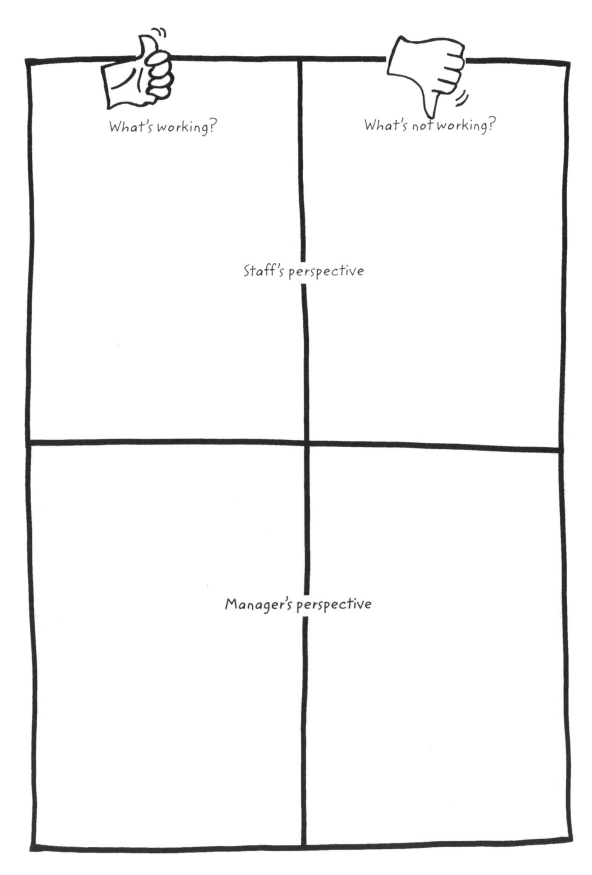

Figure 6.2 Working/not working from staff and manager's perspectives

They each bring their top three things that are working and the top three things that are not working to discuss at their supervision meeting.

At the meeting, the team leader and staff member review what each person has written and ask clarifying questions to make sure they understand each other's perspective. Starting with items that are working, as the team leader, ask if there is anything that needs to be done to ensure that these continue or increase? You might agree to some action items around supporting those areas in the future. Add these to the performance development support plan.

Then look at items that are not working and talk about what success would look like if these areas were working really well. Agree to actions and clear performance expectations to move in the direction of success. You can use tools you have learned in previous chapters, like the Doughnut tool, or the Expectation Arrow, to clarify expectations and performance standards. Actions that emerge can be added to the performance development action plan, which we shared in Chapter 4.

Reflect on the person's one-page profile. Have either of you learned anything about what is important to the person, or how they want to be supported as part of this process? As a team leader, have you noticed anything that could be added to the appreciation section of their one-page profile?

FIVE WAYS TO WELL-BEING

The New Economics Foundation[50] identified five evidence-based actions (adapted for teams and organisations) that lead to individual well-being:

1. Connect: With people you support, employees, funders, like-minded organisations and community partners in the boardroom or meetings, lunchroom, grocery store and the local movie theatre. Building connections wherever opportunity exists will bring riches you could not have anticipated.

2. Be active: Start a lunchtime walking group. Play ping-pong. Do yoga. Get a ten-minute massage. Enter a team in the local softball league. Have fun with Karaoke in the break room. Exercise and laughter will make you feel healthy and happy – discover the joy of playing together while working together.

3. Take notice: Listen. Seek to understand. Notice the talents and contributions of others. Give praise and appreciation. Reflect on what is important to people on your team and the people you support. Know thyself. Be aware of the external environment and how it impacts on your organisation.

4. Keep learning: Reflect on what you have tried, what you have learned, what you're pleased or concerned about, and what you'll do next based on what you have learned. Read, then read some more. Learn how to lead. Take on a different responsibility. Tackle a new computer application. Stretch yourself; find a coach, learning new things is fun. It will make you more confident and can give you a competitive edge.

5. Give: Thank volunteers. Smile on the phone. Celebrate your customers. Support your staff. Join a networking group. Collaborate with other organisations around a common goal. Share resources. Donate your time and expertise to support a community event. Let staff participate in community service as a company benefit. Create a board-giving policy.

You can use person-centred thinking tools to help learn about how your team are doing on each of these areas, and where they can improve. Michelle describes how the team decided to use the headings from *Five Ways to Well-Being* to explore what was important to them in relation to connecting, taking notice, learning, giving and being active. Michelle said:

We paired up and had conversations about each area, then created personal action plans that ensured that we were taking care of ourselves and each other as team members. One of the key learning points for Vicky, as she is self-employed, was that it was all too easy to let work encroach on time with her family during the evenings and weekends, and on holiday. Using the Five Ways helped Vicky to highlight what was no longer working for her, to clarify what mattered to her and to address this in her action planning.

Table 6.2 *Vicky's Five Ways to Well-Being*

Home	What is important to you about this?	How are you doing now?	What do you want to change?	Actions
Connect.	To spend quality time with my family doing things which are fun and outdoors. Seeing my friends at least once a week. Speaking to my parents on the phone or Skype at least four times a week. Keeping in contact with friends and family who live far away via Facebook or text.	We don't get the opportunity every week to spend quality time together due to work, homework, exams, etc. We always eat together. I always have time off over school holidays to spend with the children. I don't see my friends as often as I would like, but we do phone and text. I keep in touch with friends and family who live away in a way I am happy with.	Not to book work in for a Monday which often means that I have to travel on a Sunday, our only family day. Not to do administrative work in the evening so that we can have some time together if possible.	I will not book work in on a Monday which means that I have to travel on a Sunday. I will not do work during the evening when at home. I will take opportunities to do this when I'm away.
Be active.	To go for a walk as often as I can, at least half an hour four times a week. Once a week to go for a long walk on my favourite beach, Porthdinllaen.	If I am at home, I will go for a walk every day, weather permitting! I enjoy a walk in the morning as it sets me up for the day. We will go for a long walk on a Sunday, often to the beach. If I am away at work, I will try to find a shopping centre to walk around.	I would like to find a way to exercise when I'm away, although I don't like to go out on my own, so I will not go for a walk. I would like to be more active in my community, but find it hard to commit to anything as I am often away with work.	I will download my Davina DVD onto my laptop, so I can do some exercises while I am away. I will look into what activities are available in my local community which do not require constant commitment.

cont.

Home	What is important to you about this?	How are you doing now?	What do you want to change?	Actions
Take notice.	I love the sea and the mountains and really appreciate where I live. Just going on my usual morning walk allows me to see Snowdon and the sea.	I am happy that I can see the things that I love every day. It helps me to relax and put things in perspective.	Being able to spend more time outside.	I will go for a walk every day I am at home.
Keep learning.	To keep learning as a mum, how to support my children well as they grow up into young adults. Skills of diplomacy and negotiation are important to allow them to grow, to keep them safe and for me to feel happy. I love cooking, so to be able to learn new skills in the kitchen and learn to cook new dishes helps me to relax. I love to learn new skills, but my work is keeping me busy enough in that respect.	I am learning not to be as anxious and to let my eldest child be more independent, which is a struggle for someone who likes to be in control! I do cook and I buy *Good Food* magazine every month and try new recipes all the time.	To be more relaxed and prepared to allow my eldest child in particular to grow up and become independent. That I don't buy any more magazines as my cupboard is full to overflowing.	I will aim to book a cooking weekend with Rick Stein in the next 12 months. I will stop buying *Good Food* magazine and download it onto my iPad instead. I will download the March copy onto my iPad.
Give.	I like to give to my community and have in the past been very active, particularly with our local primary school.	Not very well now. I have stopped helping with a number of clubs, etc., as my children have gone to a different school and work means that I cannot commit to things as I may be away.	I would like to find a way to contribute that means that I wouldn't let anyone down if I couldn't attend something.	I will find out if there is anything in my local community that I could contribute to which doesn't require weekly attendance.

The team found that other person-centred thinking tools can drill down into particular areas. For example, thinking about the 'connecting way to well-being':

- You could use a relationship circle to look at who is in your life at the moment, and what you could do to develop the relationships you have already.

- You could use community mapping to show where you spend your time and where you're connected.

- You could include other places you want to be, and how you'd like to be a part of your community.

- You could use *presence to contribution* as a way to plan your steps to be involved more in your community.

- You could use the *working/not working* tool around your connections.

- You could use *four-plus-one* person-centred thinking tool to reflect on what you've been trying to be more connected to.

In the chapter so far we have shown how these person-centred practices are used with individuals. They are also powerful at a team level, to reflect on progress, in particular the *four-plus-one questions*. *Working/not working from different perspectives* is embedded in the person-centred team review process, and how we can aggregate information from what's working/not working through the *Working Together for Change* process.

LEARNING LOGS FOR TEAMS

Earlier we introduced *learning logs* as a way to reflect on individual support. The following is an example of how they can be used by a team:

> A team of person-centred thinking trainers used a *learning log* to capture their experiences delivering a new curriculum. Individual trainers added stories about different ways of delivering content and engaging participants. Then they posted the *learning log* online for all trainers to access, which became a very useful resource for trainers who were looking to continue to improve their delivery in the classroom.
>
> The training team meets quarterly and reviews any additions to the *learning log*. As a team they consider the significance of the learning, and use the insights to agree to future changes to the training content.

PERSON-CENTRED REVIEWS

Person-centred reviews can take place around an individual the team supports, and as a team reviewing their own performance.

In the Performance chapter we shared the process and information from John's person-centred review, and how this focused the team on what they needed to do to enable John to achieve his outcomes. Figure 6.4 is a graphic that summarises that process.

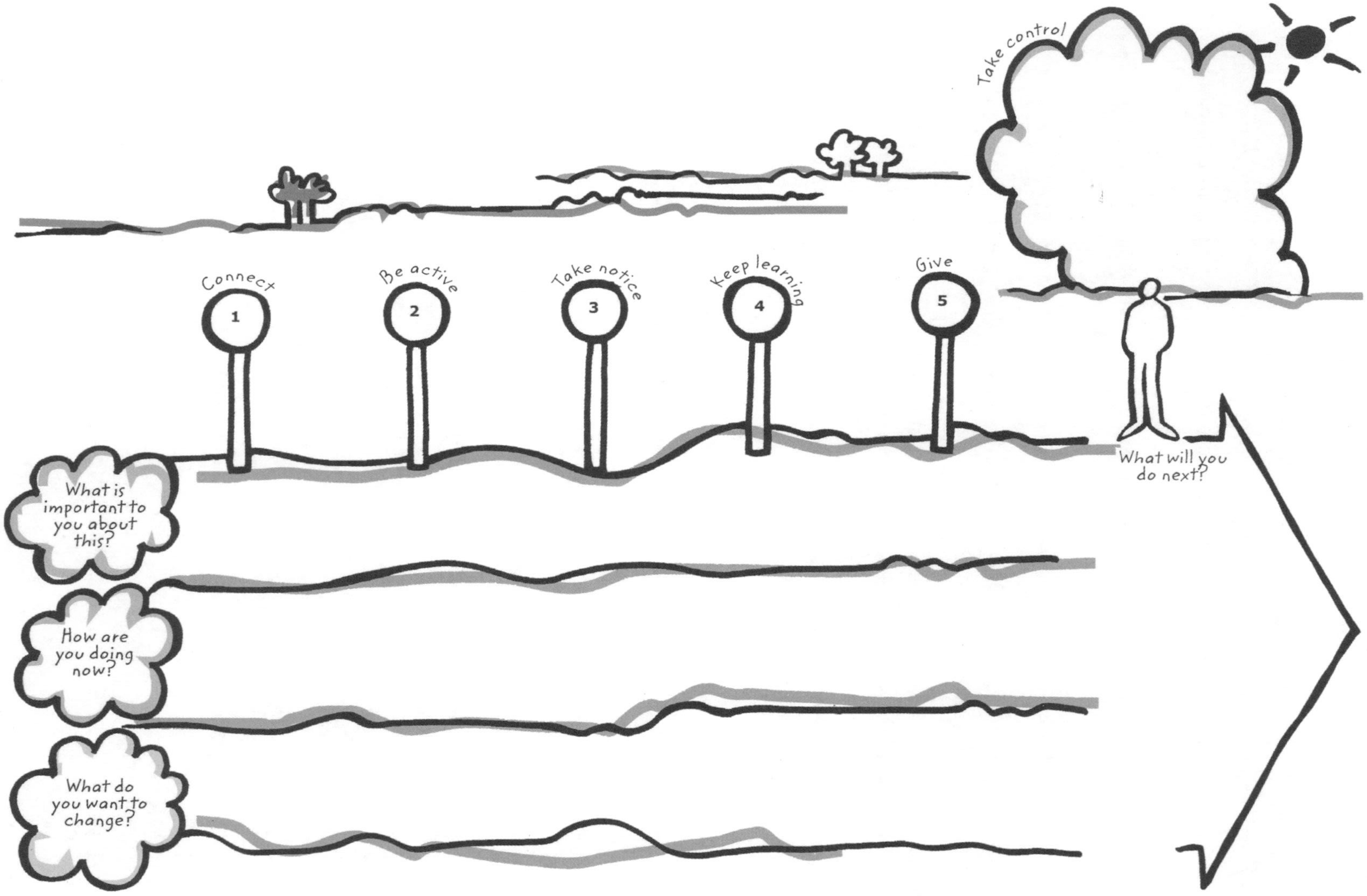

Figure 6.3 Five Ways to Well-Being

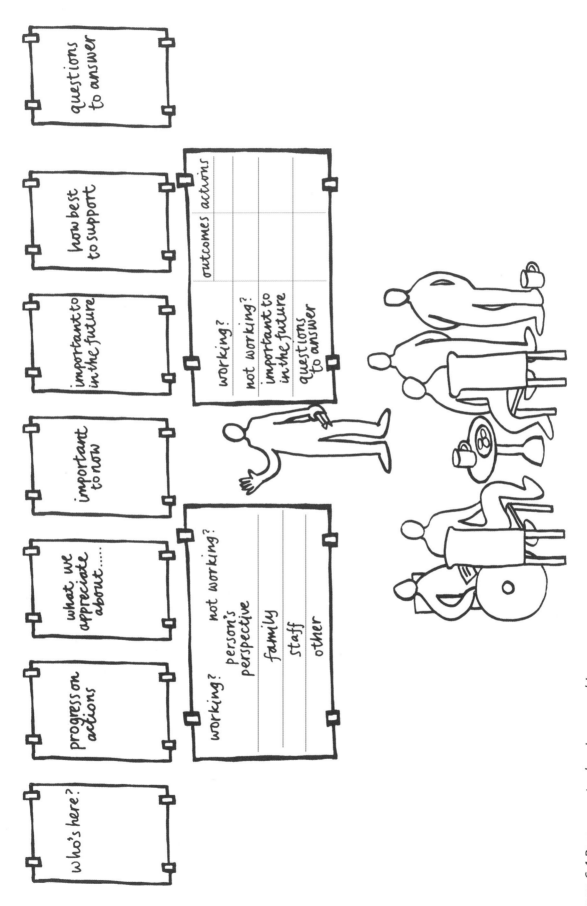

Figure 6.4 *Person-centred reviews graphic*

Imagine, Act and Succeed (IAS) is a Manchester-based registered charity that can offer support in learning disabilities, transition, self-direction support and individual service funds. Ruth Gorman, an experienced trainer and CEO of IAS, saw the potential of using person-centred reviews for teams. Now each team does an annual self-assessment as well as using the process with each employee the organisation supports. Ruth says:

> The introduction of the person-centred review process has changed the culture of the organisation. It is a fantastic way to use common language for all connected to IAS.
>
> Using person-centred reviews in teams to review what is important to the team and what is working and not working from different perspectives, has resulted in better working relationships, a clearer understanding about the direction of each team in the organisation and their commitment to our statement of purpose.
>
> We continue to develop our thinking in this area by introducing the person-centred review process for all staff, rather than an appraisal. This "work review" is based on the same headings and it enables people really to focus on what they are contributing to the lives of the people we support and how they are engaging with their team and the organisation.

Here is how the questions used in a person-centred review are adapted to be used within a team:

Table 6.3 *Headings for person-centred reviews*

Headings used in a person-centred review	Headings used in a team review
What do we appreciate about the person?	What do we appreciate about our team?
What is important to the person now?	What is important to us as a team now?
What is important to the person for the future?	What is important in the future?
What does the person need in order to stay healthy, safe and to be supported well?	What support does our team need to do our best work and deliver our purpose? From each other? From the manager? From others?
What questions do we need to answer?	What questions do we need to answer? What do we still need to figure out?
What is working/not working from different perspectives?	What is working/not working from different perspectives? From each team member? From the manager? This is done specifically around the team's performance outcomes and how the team works together.

Similar to person-centred reviews around individuals, a person-centred team review ends with specific performance targets or outcomes for the upcoming year and actions to achieve them.

GENERATING TEAM ACTIONS DURING A TEAM REVIEW BY REFLECTING ON THE FIVE PS

During a person-centred team review at Tri-Counties Regional Center, service co-ordinators looked at what was working/not working within the team. Mary Beth placed the person-centred team headings – purpose, people, performance, process and progress – on the grid to encourage breadth and depth in their responses.

Offering these prompts as a way to think about what was working/not working allowed for deeper thinking and a more thorough review of all aspects of the team.

After all ideas were recorded, they looked for common themes, which were used to prioritise top goals and generate action items.

While some of the generated action items related to providing direct service co-ordination to people, others addressed internal relationship or organisational process issues that were preventing the team from doing its best work. Having the input organised in that way helped the team develop a comprehensive set of actions.

WORKING TOGETHER FOR CHANGE (WTFC)[51]

WTFC is a collaborative, eight-stage process that takes person-centred information from reviews, or what is working/not working, and uses it to inform strategic change. It's been used in schools, by the Department of Health, and in adult health and social care, and is now being used instead of staff satisfaction questionnaires by some providers.

Using the process instead of questionnaires involves taking anonymous information from staff one-to-ones or appraisals about what is working/not working, then a group of staff and managers clusters that data to identify common themes. Managers and staff agree on strategic actions to ensure that what is working continues into the future.

Theming what isn't working can reveal main areas of discontent within staff across the organisation. The process includes ways to understand why it's happening, and the group then agrees on success indicators about each theme. Once there are clear indicators, the group decides on strategic actions to change what isn't working and move towards those things that can work

Friends of the Elderly is a charity dedicated to supporting older people. Redcot Care Home is one of 14 residential services and is home to 32 people, providing 24-hour support for residents. Redcot is staffed by support workers, volunteers and medical professionals.

The staff team used WTFC to reflect on what is working/not working in the context of the success statements in the organisation's strategy. Friends of the Elderly's one-page strategy states success for staff as:

- We are listened to and share a sense of belonging.

- We are empowered to feel confident and competent.

- We are able to contribute to people's lives.

- We support the homes, services and success of the organisation.

Information about what was working/not working in relation to those statements was gathered from each staff member, clustered and themed. It was very encouraging to hear what they thought was working well:

- I can really rely on other staff.

- Good working relationship with other staff.

- Good staff team who back each other up.

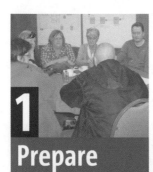

1 Prepare

Agree how, when and where you want to use Working Together for Change and who needs to be involved. Ensure people have a recent person-centred or outcomes focused review.

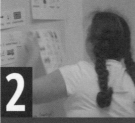

2 Collect

Gather the information from reviews – what are the two top things that are working and not working for each individual, and what do they want for the future?

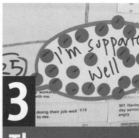

3 Theme

Work with a range of stakeholders, including people with support needs, to recognise themes in the information from reviews and give each theme an "I" statement.

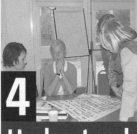

4 Understand

Work together to understand the root causes of what is not working for people and prioritise the top ones to address.

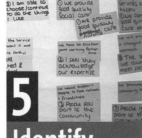

5 Identify Success

Identify what success would look like if the root causes were addressed and changed. Agree success statements from different perspectives.

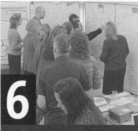

6 Plan

Look at what is happening already to move towards success, think together about a range of other ways to make change and agree which ideas to turn into action plans.forward.

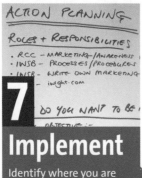

7 Implement

Identify where you are now (baseline) and how else you will know you've been successful (indicators). Share this information and start to implement action plans.

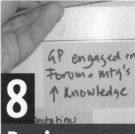

8 Review

Evaluate progress against success criteria and write Working Together for Change report. Communicate progress and next steps to all involved and other people interested in the changes.

Figure 6.5 Working Together for Change – an eight-step process

When they looked at the statements about what wasn't working, communication came out as a top theme. Here are some statements people made:

- Communication isn't consistent.

- Not notifying change of policy.

- Lack of communication.

- Poor communication between senior care staff. One says one thing, another says something different.

- The way we record on a daily basis – we don't record some things.

- Seniors give confusing/conflicting messages.

The next step was to identify root causes, and what team success would look like. From this, the group developed ideas for actions that became specific and measurable.

Table 6.4 Identifying root causes and what success looks like

What's not working	Root cause	What success would look like	Actions
Inconsistent communication.	Seniors have different ideas of what/how things should be done. Seniors not working to a consistent framework.	Team communication is excellent. We all have the same messages and information.	Seniors to have regular meetings. Seniors to have a framework of procedures to work to. Seniors to listen to suggestions from health care assistants.

ADDRESSING POOR PERFORMANCE

We've shared a range of ways to look at individual and team performance. So what happens when you discover poor performance? You would start with a clear understanding of why this has happened and address the issues differently, depending on the cause. Here are some possible causes and solutions:

- If the person didn't fully comprehend what was expected of them, go back to the Doughnut, look at core responsibilities and where they can use their creativity, and see if these need further clarification.

- If the person didn't get the support they needed, look at what good support looks like in their one-page profile. Is it clear enough? Is it reasonable? Is it being acted on?

- If the person does not have the skills to deliver, do you have the right match between their strengths and the tasks? Or do you need to help them improve their level of competency?

When Lara Harding, the People Programs Specialist at Google (voted the best place to work in the UK in 2008; and quoted in *The Happiness Manifesto* by Henry Stewart),[52] was asked what they do when someone is underperforming, she said, 'We coach and mentor the hell out of them.' So that is where to start based on a thorough understanding of why.

Progress question 2: how can we improve?

Again, as with the first progress question, we address this at both an individual and an organisational level. At an individual level this takes us into the realm of coaching. There are many excellent books on coaching, so we share one example of a process to illustrate how important coaching is as a role for a team leader.

The person-centred practices that we have already mentioned in the earlier sections each result in actions for improvement. Improving as a team takes us to action planning from different directions, and *Working Together for Change*. Both of these bring together how are we doing and how can we improve, in the same way that person-centred reviews do.

TO GROW MODEL

Coaching is a person-centred approach that can influence the team's learning culture. It is an ongoing process of inquiry with the purpose of helping individuals to achieve their desired goals.

A coaching approach allows the person being coached to direct the content and the solution. It provides the structured support and feedback for individuals to feel more competent and confident when applying newly learned skills, knowledge or practice. The coaching process is a vehicle to listen, understand and move the action forward.

Coaching can be introduced by a supervisor, team leader or peer. By allowing the solution to emerge in a way that makes sense for the person receiving coaching, this process keeps that person at the heart of the issue, and is a powerful process tool to engage and empower team members.

For those new to coaching, a good place to start is by using the *To GROW model*.

This model is very effective during a coaching conversation between team members, or between a supervisor and employee where a new skill is being learned and the employee is looking to achieve a behaviour change or performance improvement.

The *To GROW model* is straightforward as it focuses on a measurable goal, the review of possible options and the development of an action plan. The *To GROW model* is similar to a travel agent planning a vacation:

- First, the customer decides they're going to take a vacation (their **T**opic).

- The agent helps them decide where they are going (their **G**oal).

- The agent establishes their current resources and budget (their **R**eality).

- Together they explore various ways of making the trip (their **O**ptions).

- In the final step (the **W**ill), the agent ensures that their customer is committed to making the trip and is prepared for the conditions and obstacles they may meet during their journey.

At each of these steps you can ask open-ended questions to allow the person you're coaching to share their thoughts, ideas and possible ways forward (their travel). The steps aren't always sequential, so they might bounce back and forth as new thoughts emerge.

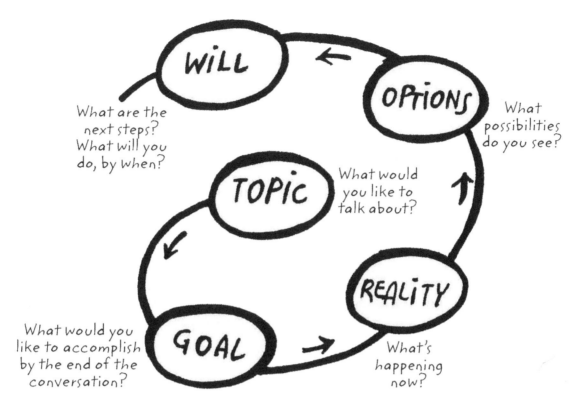

Figure 6.6 To GROW model

FOUR-PLUS-ONE QUESTIONS

Here we move from how individuals can develop their performance to ways teams can accomplish this. The *four-plus-one questions* can be used in team meetings to review and reflect on learning and decide what to do next based on that learning.

Tell team members before a meeting that you'll be using these questions so they can come prepared. You can write their ideas on a flipchart and ask them to write down their answers as they arrive at the meeting, or use sticky notes to facilitate groupings of similar ideas. This is an efficient way to ensure that everyone's views inform new actions.

Four-plus-one questions

Information-gathering

1. What have we learned?

2. What have we tried?

3. What are we pleased about?

4. What are we concerned about?

Creating action steps

5. What will we do next based on what we've learned?

   Teresa, Dana, Vivian and Greg were exploring ways to improve their team's planning process. Teresa was the Director of Services and supervised Dana, a department manager. Vivian and Greg were support staff who reported directly to Dana.

When they started talking about what kinds of changes could be implemented, Teresa and Dana dominated the conversation. Dana knew Vivian and Greg had great ideas on the topic, but noticed they were silent during the meeting.

She said, 'I'm concerned that we're dominating the conversation and we're not hearing from everyone. Is it okay if we try having this conversation in a different way?'

With the group's permission, Dana placed four sheets of paper in the middle of the table and gave a stack of sticky notes to each person. She asked the group, 'As we think about our goal to improve our planning process, what have we tried?'

She asked everyone to write their ideas on the sticky notes and put them on the first piece of paper. The group reviewed all the notes and moved on to the next question, 'What have we learned?' They completed these steps for all four questions, clarifying responses as they went through the process.

Then they each wrote their responses to the plus-one question, 'What should we do next based on what we've learned?' The results were remarkable. Through this process the group arrived at steps that were very different from those Teresa and Dana had originally proposed.

All team members were engaged and involved, despite the power differential in the room. The end result was much better because everyone benefited from all the information collected on the sticky notes. Using this structure they were able to discuss clearly the issue and arrive at action steps in about 15 minutes.

WORKING TOGETHER FOR CHANGE (WTFC)

Both *Working Together for Change* and the multi-level action planning used at Tri-Counties ensure that other stakeholders can contribute to the reviewing of progress and developing performance objectives.

How effective are patient satisfaction questionnaires as a way for patients to give feedback on a team's performance? Isn't it fair to say that, too often, questionnaires are quantitative, box-ticking exercises that lack the depth or power to influence real change?

At Bispham Hospital, a 40-bed rehabilitation unit near Blackpool run by Spiral Health, the staff team use *Working Together for Change (WTFC)* to gather meaningful, qualitative feedback from patients – and to work with patients to review the team's performance, analyse issues and set objectives for improvement.

The team at Bispham Hospital are managers, healthcare assistants, therapists (occupational therapists and physiotherapists), non-executive directors, and nurses. A representative group from this team spent a day using the WTFC process.

Cheryl Swan, the unit's Clinical Director, met with each patient individually. She asked each person for two things that are working, two things that are not working and two things that people would like to see in the future, if they were to come back to the unit again. Cheryl's approach to the interviews was very personal. She told patients, 'We want to make your experience here a good one for you. We don't just want you to do a survey, we want you to tell us in your own words what is working while you've been here and what is not working.'

The statements gathered were transferred onto coloured cards to make the information easier to cluster and theme, then the assembled group worked together to sort through all the cards. The green cards represented things that patients considered were 'working' in the unit and there were many positive comments about the staff. Patients said, 'You can't fault the staff,' and 'The staff are excellent, they are always there for you.' They also commented that they were feeling confident, strong and calm during their stay.

The group then turned to the red cards, which themed what was 'not working'. The largest group of cards reflected the issue that the food was unpopular. In the next largest group, patients were asking for more demonstrations of their exercises. Patients also commented that, 'It took too long for people to come to me,' and 'I was hurried to meals but then I had to wait,' Finally, the group looked at the three blue cards that represented what people wanted to see in the future. The suggestions were that the unit should have a large TV screen for the short-sighted, that an internet station would be useful and that the unit should know more about patients prior to their arrival.

By now the group was on stage four of the process, during which the objective was to understand all the comments from the perspective of all stakeholders in the hospital. The group felt that the top issues of concern were the food, the feeling that patients were being hurried to dinner but then having to wait to be served, and that it took too long for staff to come to patients when bedside buzzers were rung. The group took each issue in turn and looked at what the root causes could be.

The group was divided according to role – patients, staff (therapists and nurse) and managers – and each group was asked for a clear success statement. Each group's statement was similar, but the nuances that came through reflected their particular perspectives and were therefore important to note. At this point the group could start to look at actions to move towards this success.

Getting the food right was a key issue. Managers agreed to talk to the catering staff to see what could be changed that was within their control on site – and they sought, and gained, permission for staff to make gravy on site. From now, catering staff were expected to take more responsibility for the amount and quality of food they served on a plate. Evening menus were changed so that, along with sandwiches, there was a greater choice of hot dish. Finally, managers agreed that they would eat meals with patients on a regular basis. This attention to detail was repeated with each one of the main 'not working' issues raised.

Spiral Health's experience is that WTFC enables patients, nurses, managers and therapists all to make a direct and significant contribution to both changing the patient experience for the better and informing the business planning process.

If you visit the hospital, you can see a noticeboard at the entrance where the themes from WTFC are displayed, along with the new actions agreed by the group and what progress is being made on these.

ALIGNING PLANNING ACROSS THE ORGANISATION

Now let's think about how team progress and planning can align with organisational planning or strategic planning. People's typical experience of action planning is from the top down.

Downward directives come from the organisation's leadership, and teams are charged to accomplish specific objectives. Team members may have little to say about what the objectives are, but it is hoped they have more voice in how they will be implemented.

Person-centred organisations and teams seek deliberately to shift the focus of control in the planning process to include more upward and lateral input. They tend to create an environment in which determining strategy and action planning are more participatory.

- *Upward input* is generated by people who are supported by the organisation, based on what is working/not working and future wishes.

- *Lateral input* comes from within the team or across the organisation. As team members reflect on their team performance, they generate actions that relate to their internal work.

- *Action plans* must be checked for alignment with the team purpose. If they don't help the team to deliver its purpose, it must be carefully considered whether team resources should be allocated in that manner.

Alignment across the organisation is very important. Team leaders can guide staff to use the organisation's mission and team purpose statements along with any strategic goals as an anchor to develop team-level and individual performance goals.

The most effective action plans consider the input of all three perspectives – upward, downward, and lateral – that are driven by team purpose and influenced by the other four Ps (people, performance, process and progress) of a person-centred team.

Tri-Counties Regional Center (TCRC) uses a combination of input from all three perspectives to determine strategic priorities for the organisation as well as team-level and individual goals.

Upward

Each year TCRC conducts a satisfaction survey, during which people who receive services are interviewed about their personal choice and control in the planning process, their satisfaction with services, and the degree to which their needs are met. After the results are compiled, the survey administrator meets with every team manager to share and discuss team-level data. They talk about emerging themes and possible actions the team might focus on for continuous improvement.

TCRC also invites input from the person served, family members, service providers, regional centre staff and other community partners to identify emerging issues and priorities to be considered when developing a three-year organisational strategic plan.

Downward

Once all of the input is considered, the Board of Directors approves a number of strategic priorities for the organisation to act on during a three-year period.

Lateral

Using stakeholder input, satisfaction data, and board direction about strategic priorities, the teams engage in establishing annual team-level goals. With those goals in place, the process becomes easier to make sure they become part of the employee performance review process.

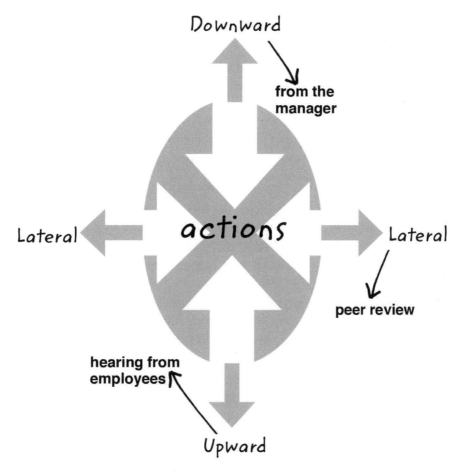

Figure 6.7 Aligning planning

In this multi-level approach, teams have autonomy in setting a direction that is aligned with the organisation's priorities, while still being accountable for performance. They contribute to the vision by adding the details.

Your team can choose things within your sphere of influence as long as you maintain organisational priorities. Other actions are generated from the person-centred team review and the input of people you support.

Getting started

You got started with the team process when you looked at performance. You looked at what success looked, felt or sounded like, and how you could know how well you're doing. In this chapter we have introduced you to a variety of ways to look at individual and team performance and well-being.

HOW DO YOU KNOW HOW YOU'RE DOING?

One place to start is to *evaluate how well you are evaluating*! Remember, you want a range of proportionate approaches. It would be wonderful to use them all in your team, but you shouldn't spend more time reviewing progress than actually doing the work.

Start by looking at the methods you use to check progress at individual and/or and team levels, and whether you're doing them around performance and well-being. Do you notice any gaps?

TRY SOMETHING NEW

Even though you may feel you already have methods for checking progress and reflecting on learning, there might be some in this chapter you could try. For instance, you could swap satisfaction questionnaires for *Working Together for Change*, or *learning logs* for progress notes.

Recording progress in the person-centred team plan

We are assuming that you already have a record of how you are recording progress in your one-page strategy or equivalent part of your person-centred team plan. Now you can either add to this or create a separate page that describes the different ways that you are using to understand how you are doing (progress question 1). When it comes to 'How can we improve?' typically you will have these recorded as new performance objectives or actions.

Figure 6.8 shows what the Oxnard Children's Team did – they added an action plan for a three-month period.

The Oxnard Team Plan graphically represented the information on an 11 x 17 inch sheet so that team members could post it in their work areas as a constant reminder of what brings them together as a team, and the work to be done in the months ahead (see Figure 6.9).

NorthStar Supported Living Services drafted their team plan using a team foundation poster and then used it to create the finished plan in Figure 6.10.

You can see that the plan includes: their purpose; information about what is important to team members; core responsibilities to describe performance; sections on process, including how to communicate and how meetings will be run; an action plan; and commitments to review and update their plan regularly.

To ensure that a plan doesn't get shelved and not used, a team needs to agree on a time for the next progress review. Team members need to be clear about the purpose and benefits of using a team plan as a road map to stay focused on and use to arrive at intended targets.

Members of the NorthStar leadership team made a list of team commitments to growing and sustaining their team plan (see Figure 6.11).

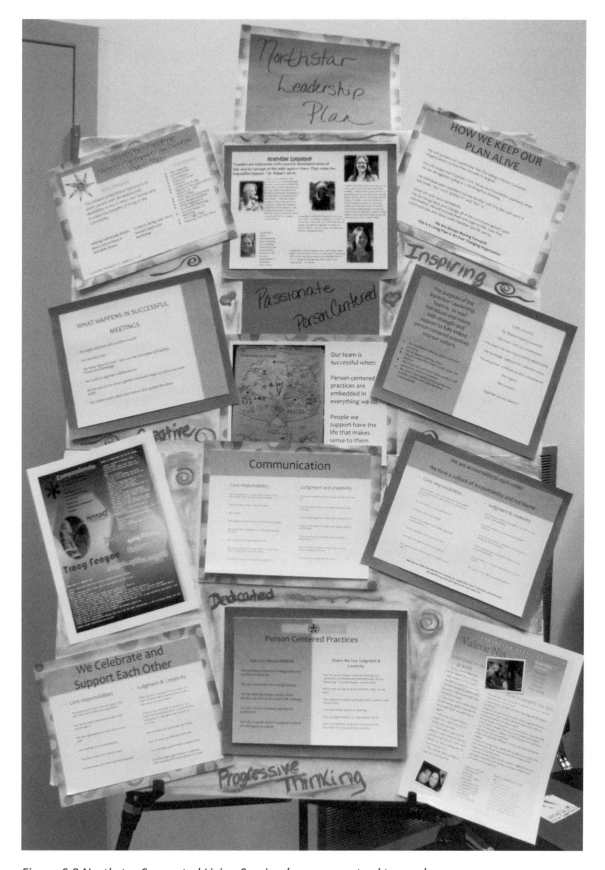

Figure 6.8 Northstar Supported Living Services' person-centred team plan

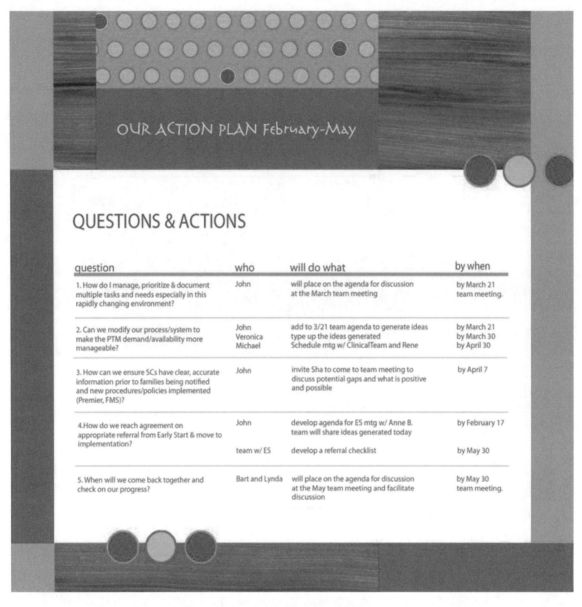

Figure 6.9 Oxnard Children's Team's person-centred team plan

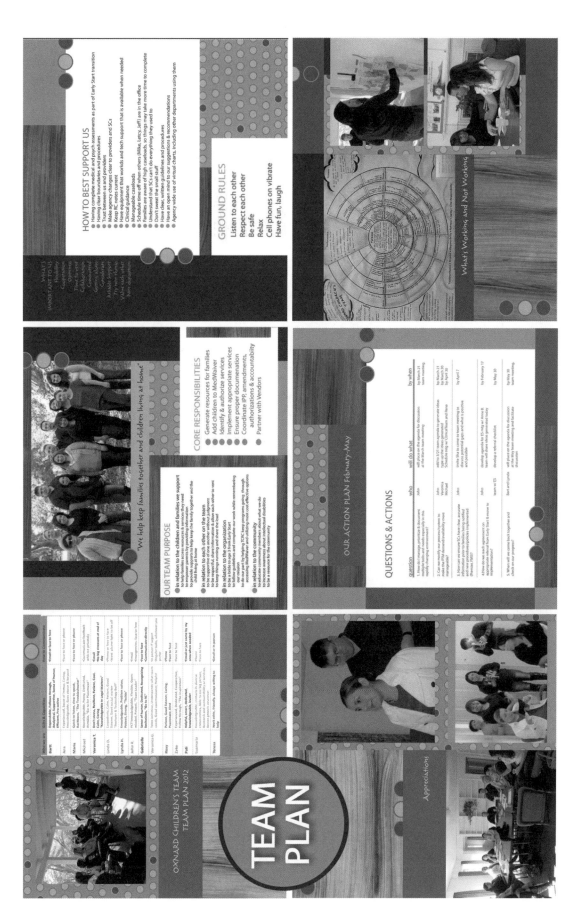

Figure 6.10 Oxnard Children's Team's three-month action plan

HOW WE KEEP OUR PLAN ALIVE

We will update our Leadership Plan (for being a Person Centered Organization) no less than annually in August.

We will review our Purpose, Core Values and Foundation quarterly when we are all together using 4+1, Working/Not Working...

As individual team members we are familiar with the plan and use it in our work: We "JUST KNOW IT" and "DO" it.

HOW WE ADD NEW MEMBERS-
We do not go back and change all of the previously agreed upon information. We will include their one page profile, how they communicate, and other team member specific pieces.

We Are Always Moving Forward!!
This Is A Living Plan In An Ever Changing Organization

Figure 6.11 Keeping the team plan alive

Progress launches you and your team back to people, performance and processes. Your purpose should not change. In Jim Collins's book, from *Good to Great*, he says that your principles should stay the same but how you achieve them will alter. However, your purpose may change over time in some organisations, for example, the paradigm in social care is evolving from delivering 'care' to 'choice and control' as personalisation becomes embedded. We are starting to see the words 'choice' and 'control' reflected in the way that organisations describe their purpose. The team who support Anne-Marie, in Chapter 4, reflect this change.

From the person-centred practices that you have seen in this chapter, we hope that the connections between the Ps are clear, and that what you learn about how well you are doing and how you can improve are likely to lead to:

- changes in the understanding of the people in your team, and how you work together. Has 'progress' led to updates to people's one-page profiles, or your team guidelines about how you work together?

- changes in your performance. Has there been any new information from stakeholders or your team about what success looks like? Have you increased your performance expectations based on this? Have you added to or amended your original ideas about how you will measure success?

- changes to your processes. By exploring what is working and not working for people, or what you have tried and learned, does this mean that any of your processes need to be tweaked or changed?

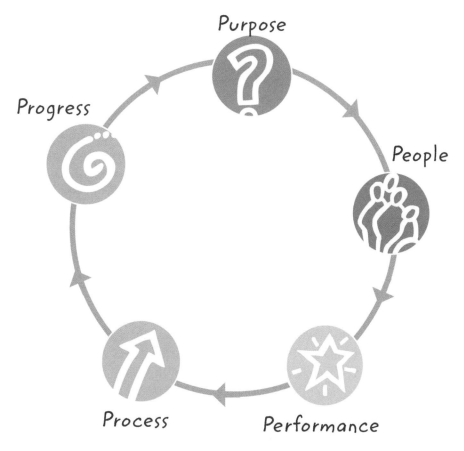

Figure 6.12 From progress and back again

Table 6.5 *Progress checklist*

Progress checklist	Strongly disagree	Disagree	Agree	Strongly agree
You have a way of evaluating individual performance and setting new targets.	☐	☐	☐	☐
You participate in regular evaluations of team performance.	☐	☐	☐	☐
You know how you can capture views of other stakeholders to know how well you're doing as a team.	☐	☐	☐	☐
Insights and next steps are recorded in the team plan.	☐	☐	☐	☐

Conclusion

> Wherever you work, your job as a manager is to make your people be the best they can be – and usually they don't know just how good they could be. It's individuals that make the difference
>
> *Alan Jones, Chairman Emeritus of Toyota UK, cited in the MacLeod and Clarke report[53]*

We hope we have shown that person-centred teams mean paying attention to both people and performance through person-centred practices, which can enable staff to feel engaged in their work and productivity.

Research shows that organisations that pay attention to employee engagement are the most successful. The MacLeod report to the UK government demonstrated the direct link between employee engagement and business results (MacLeod and Clarke 2009, *Engaging for Success: Enhancing Performance Through Employee Engagement*). In the public sector it suggests that engagement is crucial for 'driving the performance and well-being of public servants' (p.5). The research showed that engaged employees stayed longer in the organisation (were 87 per cent less likely to leave) and had less sick days.[54]

Here are drivers that lead to great employee engagement (p.33):

- Leadership which ensures a strong, transparent and explicit organisational culture which gives employees a line of sight between their job and the vision and aims of the organisation. *We are confident that a one-page strategy can achieve this.*

- Engaging managers who offer clarity, appreciation of employees' effort and contribution, who treat their people as individuals and who ensure that work is organised efficiently and effectively so that employees feel they are valued, and equipped and supported to do their job. *You can't treat people as individuals until you know them as individuals. One-page profiles enable you to match your support to the person and show that you value and recognise what matters to them.*

- Employees feeling they are able to voice their ideas and be listened to, both about how they do their job and in decision-making in their own department, with joint sharing of problems and challenges and a commitment to arrive at joint solutions. *Your person-centred team plan will record how you make sure you listen to each other and how you make decisions together.*

In the Introduction we shared 12 questions that directly relate to employee engagement and satisfaction. Let's return to them to illustrate how purpose, people, performance, process and progress and the person-centred practices related to them can contribute to your staff being able to answer yes to those questions:

How can person-centred teams contribute to employee engagement and satisfaction?

TWELVE QUESTIONS RELATING TO EMPLOYEE ENGAGEMENT AND SATISFACTION

1. Do I know what is expected of me at work?

Performance and process: (you'll see this in…)

- A one-page strategy that specifies what the team is working towards.

- A Doughnut that clarifies responsibilities in delivering success.

- Team guidelines that include what is expected of team members, and how they work together.

2. Do I have the materials and equipment to do my work right?

Performance:

- This would be addressed as part of the person-centred supervision.

3. At work, do I have the opportunity to do what I do best every day?

People and process:

- Include what they do best and enjoy doing in their one-page profile.

- Matching is the process used to match strengths and interests to team tasks, roles and people.

- This would be reviewed during person-centred supervision, and the person-centred team review.

4. In the last seven days have I received recognition or praise for doing good work?

Progress:

- We hope that as a team leader you are doing this.

- Recognising good work is a key element of progress.

- When looking at what people have done, as recorded in *learning logs*.

- In recognising the work achieved when using the *four-plus-one* tool.

- As part of what is happening when you look at what's working/not working.

5. Does my supervisor, or someone at work, care about me as a person?

People:

- Knowing you as a person is the first step, and one-page profiles accomplish that step.

6. Is there someone at work who encourages my development?

Performance and progress

- We hope this is you as the team leader.

- *Process* is addressed in how decisions are made as a team and in team guidelines.

- Person-centred supervision is the place where *performance* will primarily happen.

- Addressing *progress*, *Five Ways to Well-Being* and *To GROW* are examples of practices that focus on development.

7. Do my opinions seem to count at work?

Process and progress:

- *Process* addresses how people make decisions as a team and in team guidelines.

- In *progress* the working/not working, *Working Together for Change*, and person-centred reviews are all examples of where people's views will be addressed.

8. Does the mission/purpose of my company make me feel my job is important?

Purpose and performance:

- Team *purpose* should directly relate to the organisation's mission and purpose so that employees can see how important their job is.

- This should be clear from the success statements in the one-page strategy.

9. Are my co-workers committed to doing quality work?

Purpose, performance, process and progress:

- Having a shared idea of what quality work means happens in both *purpose* and *performance* when the team decides what success looks like.

- In *performance* they will have clarity on expectations placed on them.

- *Process* is extended to agreements about how the team works together. Person-centred supervision and reviews indicate how well co-workers are committed to delivering quality work.

10. Do I have a best friend at work?

People:

- People are more likely to find best friends at work if they have opportunities to get to know each other and have things in common.

- One-page profiles accelerate this process.

11. In the last six months has someone at work talked to me about my progress?

Performance and progress:

- Takes place in person-centred supervision and processes such as *To GROW* and *Five Ways to Well-Being*.

12. This last year have I had opportunities at work to learn and to grow?

Performance, process and progress:

- Person-centred supervision is the place to find out how the person wants/needs to learn and grow.

- By matching people to tasks and opportunities in *process*, you can make sure you're mindful of how people want to develop.

- There are specific tools like *To GROW* and *Five Ways to Well-Being* to help put this into practice.

GETTING STARTED IN ONE DAY

We have taken you step by step through creating person-centred teams, but if you feel a bit overwhelmed with all the information, here are three ways that you could get started in *one full day*. It can be helpful to have a facilitator work with you to do this if you can, so that as manager, you can contribute rather than just facilitate. As you might expect, each starts with purpose.

1. Start with a one-page person-centred team profile, then look at what is working/not working

- Work with the team to develop their purpose statement. Then support them to develop their own one-page profiles (one hour).

- Cull the information into a one-page person-centred team profile to include purpose, what is important to the team, and how best to support each other (four hours).

- Once you have the one-page team profile, do working/not working exercises from everyone's perspectives (including you as team leader) (two hours).

- Define how purpose will be delivered.

- Define how the team is supporting each other to do great work.

- Recognise what is working and see if there is anything you can do to build on it.

- Recognise what is not working, which will provide clues as to how you and the team can proceed.

Figure 7.1 looks at what might not be working, and points to the person-centred practices that could help. Plan your next steps based on this information.

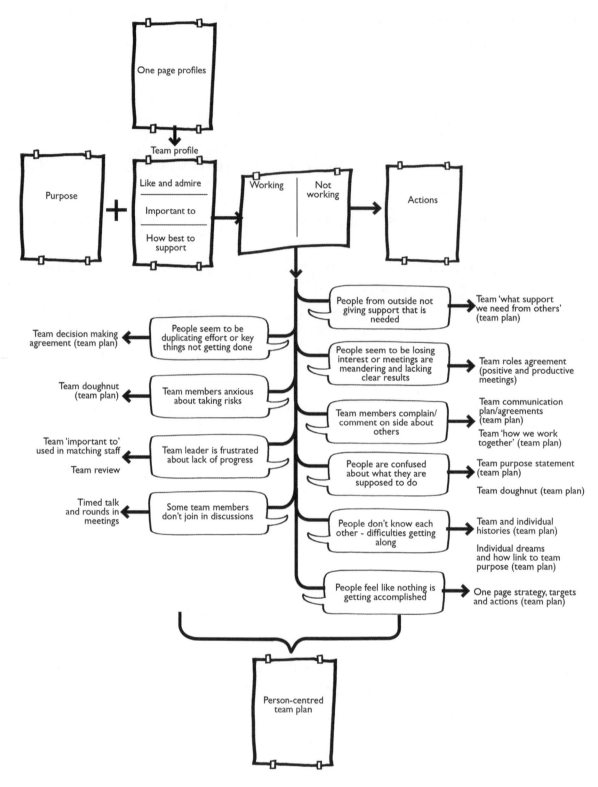

Figure 7.1 Getting Started With a Person-Centred Team Plan

2. Start with a one-page strategy

- Work with the team to develop the purpose statement (one hour).

- Look at what success looks like from different perspectives (one to two hours).

- Look at how you and the team could deliver results from each perspective, and how that can be measured (three to four hours).

Once you formulate a one-page strategy, you can develop the team's profiles to get the best match between the person and their tasks. From there you should do what's working/not working from different perspectives to decide what to prioritise next.

3. Get started with a person-centred team review

- Start by developing your team's purpose statement (one hour).

- Use the person-centred review process with the team (three to four hours) by looking at:

  - What you appreciate about the team and each other.

  - What is important to the team.

  - How to support each other.

  - What will be important in the future.

  - What is working/not working in relation to how you deliver purpose, and how you work together.

  - Questions to address within the team and issues you need to resolve.

  - How you can build on what is working, and how you can address what isn't working.

You will have enough information to start a one-page team profile (one hour), as well as actions to get started. A next step would be to develop individual one-page profiles.

Each of these ways to start generates actions and begins your person-centred team plan. If these three ways feel too much, then start with yourself. Do your own one-page profile and see how you can change your meetings, perhaps start by introducing rounds.

Person-Centred Team Self-Assessment

PURPOSE	Not implemented	Partially implemented	Fully implemented	Next steps
I know what contributions our team makes to the organisation's mission.	1	2	3	
Our team purpose was co-created with members of the team.	1	2	3	
Our team purpose was created after considering different stakeholders' perspectives.	1	2	3	
I can easily describe our team purpose to others in my own words.	1	2	3	
I am aware of my individual values and purpose and how they align with team purpose.	1	2	3	
I know how to add a purpose statement to the team plan.	1	2	3	

PEOPLE	Not implemented	Partially implemented	Fully implemented	Next steps
I know what I value and appreciate about each person in the team.	1	2	3	
I know what team members appreciate about me.	1	2	3	
I have shared and know what matters to each person in the team, and what their hobbies and interests are outside work.	1	2	3	

I am clear about what I need to know or do to support others in the team to work at their best. My team members know this about me.	1	2	3	
I know what my team members want to achieve in the future, and they know what I aspire to.	1	2	3	
I know how to complete a one-page profile and record the information in a team plan.	1	2	3	

PERFORMANCE	Not implemented	Partially implemented	Fully implemented	Next steps
I know what is expected of us as a team.	1	2	3	
I know what is expected of me as team leader.	1	2	3	
I know what team success looks like and how it will be evaluated.	1	2	3	
I know what my and the team's core responsibilities are in relation to purpose and the organisation's mission.	1	2	3	
The team accesses my individual talents and capacities to enhance performance.	1	2	3	
I have opportunities to use my individual talents and capacities to enhance team performance.	1	2	3	
We have a team plan that records our goals, objectives and success indicators.	1	2	3	
I have included my individual goals, objectives and success indicators in our team plan or on my one-page profile.	1	2	3	

PROCESS	Not implemented	Partially implemented	Fully implemented	Next steps
I understand the formal/informal team 'rules'.	1	2	3	
I know how to use *Positive and Productive Meetings* practices, including rounds and agenda development.	1	2	3	
I know how to use a person-centred supervision meeting map.	1	2	3	
I know how decisions are made in our team.	1	2	3	
I know how I will be involved in decisions that affect me.	1	2	3	
I know how to use person-centred approaches to create a learning culture for problem solving.	1	2	3	
I consider different perspectives when handling conflict.	1	2	3	
I am able to convert conversations to action steps.	1	2	3	
I know how to add process information to a team plan.	1	2	3	

PROGRESS	Not implemented	Partially implemented	Fully implemented	Next steps
People on my team know how their work will be evaluated.	1	2	3	
I have a way of evaluating my own performance.	1	2	3	
I participate in regular evaluation of our team's performance.	1	2	3	
I know how to use person-centred approaches to gather input from others when problem solving.	1	2	3	
Insights and next steps are clearly recorded in the team plan.	1	2	3	
I know what needs to be communicated and how to do it.	1	2	3	
I have added our commitments about progress to the team plan.	1	2	3	

About the Authors

Mary Beth Lepkowsky has been building internal capacity of emerging leaders, front-line supervisors, middle managers and organisation executives for more than 30 years. As Founder and Principal Consultant of Pathways Facilitation Services, Mary Beth provides leadership training, facilitation, continuous improvement and strategic planning support for non-profit and public sector organisations. She is also Assistant Director of Training and Organizational Development of Tri-Counties Regional Center, a California non-profit that provides person and family centred supports and services for individuals with intellectual and developmental disabilities. She is a certified trainer of the international Learning Community for Person Centered Practices and a Certified Professional Coach. Mary Beth lives with her husband and two sons in Solvang, California.

Helen Sanderson has led the development of person-centred thinking and planning in the UK over the last 15 years. Helen was the Department of Health's expert advisor on person-centred approaches to the Valuing People Support and Putting People First Teams. She co-authored the first Department of Health Guidance on person-centred planning and the 2010 guidance 'Personalisation through person centred planning'. Helen has worked in health, as an Occupational Therapist and then in social care for over 25 years.

Helen is the primary author of *People, Plans and Possibilities: Exploring Person Centred Planning* (1997), the first book on person centred planning in the UK, emerging from three years' research. Her PhD is on person centred planning and organisational change and she has written over 15 books on person-centred thinking, planning, community and personalisation.

Helen leads HSA, an award winning international development agency passionate about how person-centred thinking and planning can create person-centred change and contribute to changing people's lives, organisations and communities. She is Director Emeritus of the International Learning Community for Person-Centred Practices and has provided consultancy in Europe, Canada, Japan, Australia and America.

Helen lives in Heaton Moor, with Andy and her three daughters, Ellie, Laura and Kate, together with a dog, cats, hens and rabbits. She is a black belt in karate, but is now trying to spend more time doing yoga, and is learning mindfulness.

Endnotes

1. Birkinshaw, Professor J., London Business School. As cited in *The Happiness Manifesto*. Available at www.happy.co.uk/wp-content/uploads/Happy-Manifesto1.pdf., p. 7.

2. As cited by Stewart H. in *The Hidden Costs of Overbearing Bosses* by Hamel G., Lab Notes, Issue 14 December 2009, London Business School Mlab, p. 9.

3. Buckingham, M. and Coffman, C. (1999) *First, Break All the Rules*. New York, NY: Simon & Schuster.

4. Drexler, A., Sibbet, D. and Forrester, R. (1994) *The Team Performance Model*. San Francisco, CA: The Grove Consultants International.

5. HR Review, 11 November 2009. As cited in *The Happiness Manifesto*, p.117.

6. Figliuolo, M. (2011) *One Piece of Paper: The Simple Approach to Powerful, Personal Leadership*. San Francisco, CA: Jossey-Bass (imprint of John Wiley & Sons).

7. Women's History, Selected Marian Wright Edelman quotations. Available at http://womenshistory.about.com/od/quotes/a/marian_edelman.htm

8. Maloney, D. (2012) *The Mission Myth*. San Diego, CA: Business Solutions Press.

9. OASIS provides social, educational and cultural opportunities and services aimed at encouraging all adults, especially those 50 years of age and older, to become involved in preserving and improving their quality of life. Their programmes and services are administered through the Luis Oasis Senior Center in California.

10. Pavlina, S. Personal Development for Smart People. Available at http://StevePavlina.com., accessed 8 November 2013

11. Cited in MacLeod, D. and Clarke, N. (22 July 2009) *Engaging for Success: Enhancing Performance Through Employee Engagement*, p. 5.

12. Collins, J. (2001) *Good to Great*. New York, NY: HarperCollins, p.13.

13. Plas, Jeanne M. (1996) *Person-Centered Leadership: An American Approach to Participatory Management*. Thousand Oaks, CA: Sage Publications, Inc.

14. Tennant, D. *Employee Engagement Seen as Top Work Force Management Challenge*. Available at IT Business Edge: www.itbusinessedge.com/cm/blogs/tennant/employee-engagement-seen-as-top-work-force-management-challenge/?cs=50393, accessed on 9 May 2012.

15. Macey, W. H. and Schneider, B. (29 February 2008) 'The Meaning of Employee Engagement.' *Industrial and Organisational Psychology: Perspectives on Science and Practice 1*(1), 3–30.

16. *American Time Use Survey* (2010) *Bureau of Labor Statistics*. Available at www.bls.gov/tus, accessed 8 November 2013.

17. Labour Force Survey 2011. Office for National Statistics. Available at www.ons.gov.uk/ons/dcp171778_232238.pdf, accessed 8 November 2013.

18. Wagner, R. and Harter, J. K. PhD (2006) *12: The Elements of Great Managing*. New York, NY: Gallup Press.

19. Buckingham, M. and Coffman, C. (1999) *First, Break All the Rules*. New York, NY: Simon & Schuster.

20. Sanderson, H. and Stirk, S. (2012) *Creating Person-Centred Organisations: Strategies and Tools for Managing Change in Health, Social Care and the Voluntary Sector*. London: Jessica Kingsley Publishers.

21. Lepkowsky, M. B., Wennergren, H. and Calderaro-Mendoza, T. (eds) (2011) *Building Capacity for Person-Centred Thinking in Support of People with Developmental Disabilities*. Santa Barbara, CA: Tri-Counties Regional Center.

22. Harter, J. K., Frank, L., Schmidt, F.L. and Keyes, C. M. L (2003). 'Well-Being in the Workplace and Its Relationship to Business Outcomes: A Review of the Gallup Studies.' In C. L. M. Keyes and J. Haidt (eds) *Flourishing: Positive Psychology and the Life Well-Lived*. Washington, DC: American Psychological Association.

23. Boyatzis, R. E., Daniel Goleman, D. and Rhee, K. S. (2000) 'Clustering Competence in Emotional Intelligence: Insights from the Emotional Competence Inventory.' In R. Bar-On and J. D. A. Parker (eds) *Handbook of Emotional Intelligence*. San Francisco, CA: Jossey-Bass.

24. Feldman, Daniel A. (1999) *The Handbook of Emotionally Intelligent Leadership*. Paonia, CO: Leadership Performance Solutions Press.

25. Lepkowsky, M. B., Wennergren, H. and Calderaro-Mendoza T. (eds) (2011). *Building Capacity for Person-Centred Thinking in Support of People with Developmental Disabilities*. Santa Barbara, CA: Tri-Counties Regional Center.

26. Helen Sanderson Associates (2011) 'Getting your balance back.' Available at www.helensandersonassociates. co.uk/blogs/helen/2011/11/17/getting-your-balance-back.aspx

27. Luft, J. and Ingham, H. (1955) 'The Johari window, a graphic model of interpersonal awareness.' *Proceedings of the Western Training Laboratory in Group Development*, Los Angeles, CA: UCLA.

28. Myers, I. B. (1995) *Gifts Differing: Understanding Personality Type*. Mountain View, CA: Davies-Black Publishing.

29. Team Foundation Graphic: Available at www.hsapress.co.uk, accessed 8 November 2013.

30. Collins, J. (2001) *Good to Great*. New York, NY: HarperCollins, p.41.

31. Maloney, D. (2012) *The Mission Myth*. San Diego, CA: Business Solutions Press, p.26.

32. Progress for Providers, 'Checking your progress in using person-centred practices (managers).' Available at http://progressforproviders.org/checklists/checking-your-progress-in-using-person-centred-practices

33. More information on Starbursting can be found at www.mindtools.com or Mind Tools Ltd, 2nd Floor, 145–157 St John Street, London EC1V 4PY.

34. As cited in *The Happiness Manifesto*, p.59.

35. Jurow, S. (1999) *Change: The Importance of Process. Innovative Use of Information Technology by Colleges*. Washington, DC: Council on Library and Information Resources, pp. 3–7.

36. Covey, S. M. R. (2006) *The Speed of Trust*. New York, NY: Free Press.

37. As cited in *The Happiness Manifesto*, p.38.

38. Mankins, M., and Davis-Peccoud, J. *Decision Insights 9: Decision-Focused Meetings*. Available at www.bain.com/publications/articles/decision-insights-9-decision-focused-meetings.aspx, accessed from Bain & Company on 7 June 2011.

39. Michael Smull and the Learning Community for Person-Centred Practices – www.learningcommunity.us.

40. Sanderson, H., George, A. and Archambault, M. (2006) *Positive and Productive Meetings Toolkit*. Stockport, UK: HAS Press.

41. Kline, N. (1998) *Time to Think: Listening to Ignite the Humand Mind*. London: Cassell Illustrated.

42. Carver, J. M., PhD (2012) *Emotional Memory Management: Positive Control Over Your Memory*. Available at www.drjoecarver.com/clients/49355/File/Emotional%20Memory.html, accessed from Joseph M.Carver, PhD on 27 May 2012.

43. Dispenza, J. (2007) *Evolve Your Brain: The Science of Changing Your Mind*. Deerfield Beach, FL: Health Communications, Inc.

44. *Facilitative Leadership: Tapping the Power of Participation* (1997) San Francisco, CA: Interaction Associates.

45. Baker, D. A. (2009) *Multi-Company Project Management: Maximizing Business Results Through Strategic Collaboration*. Plantation, FL: J. Ross Publishing, p.58.

46. Buckingham, M. and Clifton, D. O. (2005) *Now Discover Your Strengths: How to Develop Your Talents and Those of the People You Manage*. London: Simon and Schuster UK Ltd.

47. Beachcroft, D.A.C. appraisal and objective setting on behalf of the NHS Employers organisation. Available at www.nhsemployers.org/SiteCollectionDocuments/appraisal%20and%20objective%20setting_web.pdf, accessed 18 March 2013.

48. Plas, Jeanne M. (1996) Person-Centered Leadership: An American Approach to Participatory Management. Thousand Oaks, CA: Sage Publications, p.147.

49. Collins, J. (2001) *Good to Great*. New York, NY: HarperCollins.

50. New Economics Foundation (2011) *Five Ways to Well-Being*. Available at www.neweconomics.org/publications/entry/five-ways-to-well-being-new-applications-new-ways-of-thinking/, accessed 8 November 2013.

51. Bennett, S., Sanderson, H. and Stockton, S. (2012) *Working Together for Change: Citizen-led Change in Public Services*. Available at www.groundswellpartnership.co.uk, accessed 8 November 2013.

52. Harding, L. as cited by Henry Stewart in *The Happiness Manifesto*.

53. Jones, A., Chairman Emeritus of Toyota UK, as cited in the MacLeod and Clarke report available at www.bis.gov.uk/files/file52215.pdf, accessed 8 November 2013.

54. Cited in MacLeod, D. and Clarke, N. (22 July 2009) *Engaging for Success: Enhancing Performance Through Employee Engagement*, p.5.

Index